an APPETITE for GOD

Finding Strength & Vitality for Service

Scriptural Encouragement to
Nourish the Body, Soul and Spirit

Scientific Discoveries to Guide in Permanent Health and Wellness
Using Simple Tools for Success

Linda Jeffrey Ed.D.

For information on reordering and bulk orders, visit our website **www.AppetiteforGod.com**.

Printed in the United States of America
ISBN: 978-0-9849409-3-6

FIrst Principles Press
Crestwood, Kentucky

What People Are Saying

Daniel L. Akin, M.Div., Ph.D.

First Corinthians 10:31 says, "So whether you eat or drink, or whatever you do, do all to the glory of God." *An Appetite for God* is a guide to help you do just that. Read it and grow healthy for the glory of God.

Deanna Osborn, D.O.

Dr. Jeffrey's current evidence from both scripture and science proves that health is within reach. Medical research clearly points toward clean fresh foods and supplements to nourish the body at the cellular level. The chronic illnesses I see in my practice are avoidable by following the day-to-day guidance in this book! Dr Jeffrey understands what it takes to get ones health back on track as she herself has done a remarkable job of accomplishing this.

Carroll Parish, N.D.

I enjoyed reading *An Appetite for God*. I think it is fantastic. I will be recommending it to my patients as soon as it is published. It is the most complete, instructive, and encouraging book on the subject that I have read.

Brenda McCall

Before I started my healthy living journey, my life was spiraling out of control. I had numerous health issues, depressed, fatigue, I was heavily medicated and simply hated the woman I saw in the mirror. I desperately wanted to know why my life had come to this. I needed answers, but not in a pill form. When I decided to take on the challenge of eating clean, I cut out all of the junk and replaced it with good nutritious foods, a healthy detox program, and the right supplements. I learned that all of my issues were related to food, even my depression. I've been living the healthy living lifestyle since June, 2011. I've lost 50 lbs, but I've gained so much in understanding. I now understand what foods have an adverse reaction on my body. I am no longer medicated. I have more energy than ever before and I love the woman I see in the mirror. I truly believe, as a society, we no longer understand just how good our body was created to feel.

Jill Urwick

I honestly thought that eating clean was going to be difficult to do consistently. But, it has been the most rewarding thing I have EVER done! Not only have I thoroughly ENJOYED eating the amazing meals using this plan (my family has, too)! I now make taking care of myself a priority...eating clean, exercising, etc. I plan my day around MY NEEDS rather than letting my day get in the way of that...because I'm worth it!

Vicky Jo Mantonya Church

I am totally amazed at the results I have gotten with the 40 Day Online Fitness Program. I was in a group that started Dec 1, 2013. I lost 15 pounds the first month – even through the holidays. I have continued the program for 5 ½ months and have lost over 42 pounds. I now weigh 10 pounds less than when I graduated high school. If anyone had told me I could have these results last fall I would have thought they were lying to me. This is the best thing I have ever done for myself with the exception of accepting Jesus Christ as my personal Savior.

Acknowledgments

I want to give a special thanks to the six hundred people who have participated in our online fitness boot camps, and provided questions and feedback that guided my thinking and research. ████████ gave us the original boot camp format, and Vicky Church enthusiastically developed additional content in the form of recipes and shopping lists.

Thanks to Anna Joy Jeffrey, my daughter, who has conquered lifelong obesity, and joyfully reminds people what it means to walk in health in your body, soul, and spirit. She was a major contributor to the recipes section of the book.

Thanks to Kelley Carpenter and Maureen O'Donnell who pointed me to additional research in children's health, and helped me to think about health as a family lifestyle.

Thanks to Bridgette Dunman and Krista Lee who have invested hundreds of hours in this project, and whose technical expertise continue to improve its impact and distribution.

If this project were a cell, Eunice Ray would be the mitochondria. We are all grateful for her vision, endless energy, lifelong learning, zeal for health, and extraordinary abilities to make things happen. I have worked with Colonel Ron and Eunice Ray for fifteen years. It is their leadership that continues to give me the courage to fight for righteousness and justice in every area of life.

Table of Contents

Preface

What a difference one year can make! At the age of 57, I was a size 14, frumpy, fatigued, achy and feeling old beyond my years. That year, my doctor advised me to update my will and see a specialist. Arthritis had slowed my activity to the point that walking down the stairs was a major effort, and bending over to tie my shoes was impossible. I was a little concerned, but it had been so long since I had experienced health, I didn't realize how sick I was.

I believed my MD when I was told; "It's menopause,women of a certain age gain ten pounds a year as their bodies and metabolism slow down." "It's to be expected," said my chiropractor. "We'll loosen you up with weekly visits." But the adjustments didn't help.

I thought we were healthy eaters, but our family bonding all centered on food built from sugar and fat. Having been widowed three times, our family has been through many sudden changes including financial hardships, but we also have a powerful bond built by the need to be close for each other. Part of our bonding occurred when we regularly gathered together for comfort food with pies and rich desserts being a sweet specialty. Our family was known as a circle of fabulous cooks who knew how to entertain and please with food.

The beach picture is my daughter Anna Joy, for whom weight loss has been a total focus of life since the age of ten and the death of her cherished stepfather. I tended to blame her out-of-control weight on genetics—my gestational diabetes and her resulting metabolism combined had produced a size 22, 289 pound high school senior who was miserable and dangerously obese. I had no clue what to do for her. I wrote checks to every weight loss program I could, as we careened through the "lose-20-gain-30" cycle of dieting that left my precious daughter depressed and hopeless. We began talking about stomach stapling surgery.

That's when Eunice Ray talked to Anna Joy about a 30-days to Fit program, the foundation of our current 40-Day Program. The timing was bad for me. I had just left a stressful job, was launching a new writing venture, and working hard to maintain a single-mom household on a limited budget. Why was Eunice adding more stress to my life right now?! Anna Joy was persuaded by this long-time colleague and family

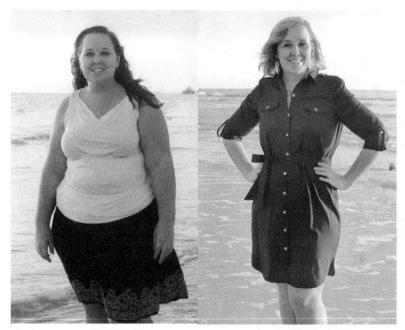

friend and really wanted to try it. My heart ached for her desperation. I agreed—but only for 30 days, and not one day longer! I loved my bread and fast food desserts after a hard day of work, and could only think I thought I was signing on to misery one more time.

I couldn't have been more wrong. With a protein shake in the morning, I was out the door in two minutes with a satisfying meal. The protein tasted great, and I realized quickly that not only was our grocery bill dropping dramatically, but the diet was so simple! We were saving much more than the cost of protein supplements because we were no longer buying processed foods.

Then a miracle happened. Around day seven of the 30 Days, I rolled out of bed and headed for the coffee as I have done for many years. At the bottom of the stairs, I screamed for Anna Joy. She came running, thinking I had fallen. "Anna Joy, I just walked down the stairs without painfully holding on to the rail!" I

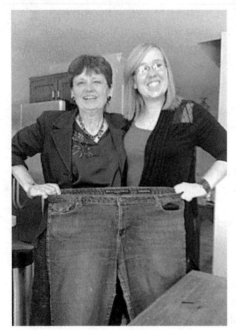

had not done that in years. Something very dramatic was happening in my body. At the end of the second week, we both did a simple seven-day cleanse, and the weight loss accelerated. I was experiencing more youthful energy, clearer thinking, and NO arthritis pain. I could get dressed without struggling to move and was beginning to realize just how sick I had been, because for the first time in years, I understood what healthy feels like!

My other daughters got on board, and when my son-in-law dropped seventy pounds, his dad and sister joined in, along with about thirty others for whom our extended family has shown the way.

We have been enjoying the 30-Days to Fit lifestyle for almost two years now. Anna Joy, who is now a beautiful size 10, calls it our 30-YEARS to fit lifestyle. Simply using a vegan protein and antioxidant rich nutrition supplements have literally transformed our family. Genetics do not control or dictate a future of hypertension, heart disease, diabetes, and cancer. We have taken control of our future health, and it is amazing, easy, affordable, and permanent. I tell everyone I meet our story and I can show you how to achieve a new level of health and wellness too.

Forward

Now therefore why tempt ye God, to put a yoke upon the neck of the disciples, which neither our fathers nor we were able to bear? Acts 15:10

The controversy of Acts 15 is about freedom in Christ. Did new converts need to keep Moses' law? Were the ceremonies that had connected people to God for centuries no longer necessary? Naturally they wanted to hold on to tradition, and so do we. In every generation the church has struggled to define salvation by grace through faith alone, and the pursuit of truth that sets men free rather than returning them again to the yoke of bondage (Galatians 5:1). The grace by which we are saved leads us to the mysterious truth of Christ's atonement, which sets us free from bondage. We are not oppressed. Our freedoms are not infringed by needless rules. There is no burden that we carry to earn salvation.

The sobering truth of Acts 15:10 is that it is not the church's job to create an atmosphere of legal boundaries that leads to the Christian life. And adding our rules and exclusions is a serious matter that puts us in danger of making God mad. Peter declared that it is "tempting God"—provoking His displeasure– to place rules on the new Gentile converts that had no bearing on their Christian faith.

It was no small decision then, when the disciples required two outward signs of an inward faith. And when you think about the gravity of making God mad, it makes it so much more important for Christians today to consider the two conditions which still applied to new converts. And surely these two would lead to freedom in Christ, since placing a yoke was so distasteful, not to man, but to God!

The two "rules" which remained for the new Gentile converts addressed food and sex. These were announced by Peter with great care, since adding rules would provoke God's wrath. But God desired so deeply to set people free in Christ, and became so angry when men took away those freedoms! Peter understood that these two areas of life must be addressed. They have the greatest potential for human bondage, and require Christians to make deliberate decisions regarding their conduct of life in order to remain free.

I never started out to devote my writing career to Peter's two issues, but that is how I have ended up here talking to Christians about their appetites. Fifteen years ago, I joined the "Restoring Social Virtue and Purity to America" campaign. As Director of Research, I examined the impact of law changes on families, and travelled the country calling state legislatures to restore the Godly moral foundations of American law. I wrote a full length monograph[1] on the history of law changes intended to disintegrate the institution of marriage while also encouraging inappropriate sexual appetites for adults and children. I have fought for my children's modesty and innocence, and for yours. Why have legislatures mandated children be bombarded with sex information in school for twelve years, when for generations, parents lovingly and safely explained the sanctity of marriage in twelve minutes? The answer is obvious. Sex outside of God's construct creates powerful bondage and so it is why Peter instructed new believers to flee from fornication, because God wants us to be free.

I am still researching and writing, and have just coauthored a natural healing handbook that details how we can improve our health position, *Dr. Deanna's Healing Handbook*[2]. A much safer, happier subject than my previous years of slug-it-out campaigning one would think, but maybe not. You see, Peter warned new believers that they must address their appetites for both food and sex if they wished to experience the

---

1   Linda Jeffrey and Ronald D. Ray. 2003. A HISTORY OF THE AMERICAN LAW INSTITUTE'S MODEL PENAL CODE: THE KINSEY REPORTS' INFLUENCE ON "SCIENCE-BASED" LEGAL REFORM 1923-2003. (Crestwood, KY: First Principles Press), available on Amazon.

2   Deanna Osborn, D.O. with Dr. Linda Jeffrey. *Dr. Deanna's Healing Handbook: Natural Aging and Disease Prevention through a Whole Foods Diet, Hormone Balance, Total Body Detox and Exercise.* Louisville: Raybonne, Inc., 2014. Available at www.deannaosborn.com.

freedom of Christ to the full. It is hard to say whether Satan has been more successful in bringing Christians to bondage through sex or food? In any case, we are bound nonetheless.

Fox News carried a report targeting Christians a few months ago entitled "Fat in Church." Yes, it seems the Church is more obese than the general population. And the problem is more sinister than overeating. We are ignorant of the greed that has driven the industrial food market to produce nutrition-depleted food with addictive properties more powerful than cocaine. That's not my opinion. It is well documented by respected men and women from the best research universities in the world. I am sad to report that today many countries will not accept American food for export because of its dangers. We are the sickest developed nation on earth. And Satan is delighted that the Church is derailed from God's Kingdom work because our minds, our bodies, and our children's generation is captured by food addictions.

I am approaching an age when I would like to repair to my home and garden to play with my grandchildren. But the truths I have found over the last 15 years are calling me to keep fighting the good fight of faith. *An Appetite for God* is the next step in obedience to Isaiah 42:22—we must cry "restore!" As I have studied the scriptures, I was guided to submit my appetites to God, and the excitement in me has grown with each step of obedience. God's people have the answers for a hungry and thirsty lost world.

He will guide us into ALL truth. I have written down the truths borne out in both scripture and science, and applied them to a 40 day program that is easy to follow, answers the why questions, and has brought astounding results. About 700 people have completed an online version of this program. Now it is finally in print form and complete as we turn to the scriptures to listen to what God says about our daily bread, and put into practice the principles of clean eating that return us to the Garden where life began.

We need to respond to Peter's admonition. Embrace your freedom in Christ, and God would have us hold on to only two principles so that we might remain free—beware of the bondage of excess in food and sex. What if the way we handle food has as much moral implication as the way we handle sex? What if the world started talking about the church as the healthiest people on earth instead of the sickest? What if you maintained your mind and body into your 80's and 90's and were still slugging away at the gates of Hell? Food cannot be the center of the Christian's world. It is simply fuel for the body, so let us bear down and find real nutrition as God intended. And once we understand the will of the Lord, we will respond as Nehemiah commanded the people—

Then he said unto them, Go your way, eat the fat, and drink the sweet, and send portions unto them for whom nothing is prepared: for this day is holy unto our LORD: neither be ye sorry; for the joy of the LORD is your strength. Nehemiah 8:10

Days 1-11
Prepping the Body

Day 1

Forty Days: A Period to Prepare for Change

All of us need to make changes in our lives, but seldom do we just wake up one day and instantaneously quit a behavior that makes life worse, or start a behavior that makes us better. Repeatedly in the Scripture forty days represents time taken to prepare for something completely new and different. Forty days as a prelude to establishing a complete change is found in a number of Biblical sites:

- Noah's ark received forty days of flooding rain—a cataclysmic event that changed the course of world history, and marked a new beginning for mankind.
- Forty days of mourning the death of Egypt's great leader, Joseph, marked the end of an era of good will for the Hebrew people and suffering ahead.
- Moses spent 40 days on Mount Sinai receiving the Ten Commandments, and a second forty days to receive them again, this time with fasting—no food or water. The Ten Commandments mark the establishment of a law order for a government with God leading his people in understanding their responsibilities toward Himself and one another.
- Caleb and Joshua scouted the land of Canaan for forty days, along with ten other spies, long forgotten for their cowardly report. They had forty days to prepare for a monumental decision as a nation—the wilderness, or the Promised Land? They chose the wilderness.
- The Israelites crouched in fear as the repulsive Philistine Goliath mocked their nation and their God—for forty days. Then David stepped forward and settled the matter.
- Elijah, famished and praying to die, received food from an angel that sustained him for forty days, a preparation time for a new mission from God.
- Jonah warned the people of Ninevah for forty days to choose between repentance and destruction.
- Jesus prepared for forty days with fasting for the temptation in the wilderness.
- Jesus remained with his followers forty days following the resurrection, and then ascended to heaven marking the beginning of the era of the Christian church.

The *Appetite for God* lessons are designed to improve the health of the body while also establishing a sense of wellbeing. The time allotment is based on the divine format of forty days. This provides time to prepare for our best service in God's kingdom by making life-preserving changes in the way we eat, cook and access our foods.

The following lessons are the result of Scripture study as well as a review of current research demonstrating that the food system is different and not necessarily nutritious. In fact, much of what passes for food today is addictive and is making us sick.

We invite you to walk in the Fit to Serve 40 Day program to make permanent health improvements and, if you are like me, you will gain a higher level of health and come out of the nutrition "wilderness". Let us joyfully join the Hebrew writer in laying aside every weight that would hinder our usefulness to the Savior. It is our intent that in these 40 days, God will transform and show you how to nourish your body because He desires to preserve your whole spirit and soul and body together (I Thessalonians 5:23).

Health Lesson:

Let's get started! The following four pages are your Getting Started Program Guide. Most of us find it easier to make changes once we understand the "why" behind it. So, the first ten days you will:

- Seek wisdom to understand God's will for our appetites for food from scripture study and prayer.
- Learn about the fundamentals of food and how it interacts with our bodies at the cellular level.
- What to do to get started, including shopping for more healthful foods.

Then we will start making food changes for good health during days 12 through 40. Each day will have a WHAT TO LEARN and a WHAT TO DO section.

During the ten days of preparation, I will outline the program's key components to give you some background knowledge on how these 40 days are going to transform you from the inside out. I'll provide you with meal plans, recipes and your grocery shopping list. It is important for you to read each daily entry and respond with your personal commitment to health. Our bodies are fearfully and wonderfully made, and also custom made—you are one of a kind. By applying principles of truth from scripture and research that has revealed God's creation, you will let go of food addictions, destructive ways of using food for comfort, and make choices for clean fuel for your mind and body.

WHAT TO DO:

- Purchase a clean protein powder supplement, free of soy and whey. We recommend pea, cranberry and rice protein.
- Read through the Getting Started pages that follow.
- Take a picture of yourself front and side. Do the mug shot thing. No one will see it unless you want them to. Get out your phone and do it. You'll be glad you did!
- Relax. You will learn as you go. Remember we have a divine 40 days for transition.

The next four pages will help you get started. We will all be on this eating program by Day 12. You can begin substituting a protein shake for a meal any time between now and then.

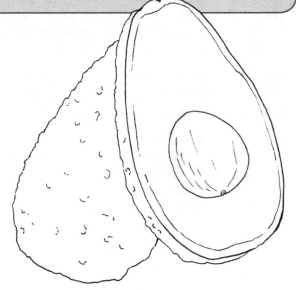

Getting Started

Breakfast

- 1/2 cup frozen fruit
- 1 cup fresh frozen spinach
- 2 scoops protein powder
- 1 scoop fiber
- 1 cup of water
- Blend in your one cup mini blender

We bought a little one cup blender, because you get out the door in the morning in under a minute when the cup is the blender and there's nothing to wash. We have used the Bella from Target, and the GE from Walmart, and the Magic Bullet. The GE mini-blender is our favorite.

Lunch

Two protein bars (recipe on page 7) with one cup of fresh berries or a Granny Smith apple. Drink plenty of water.

Dinner

4 oz. lean meat, and plenty of salad and green vegetables.

Twice a week, we added an extra carb at dinner—1/2 cup brown rice or quinoa, which will help manage carb cravings. The goal is not to be hungry. You can eat a protein bar at bedtime if hungry.

The only two oils we use are organic expeller pressed non-refined coconut oil and avocados. They add calories, but are very good for you in moderation. Don't cook vegetables in butter—they are great steamed with a dash of salt and garlic powder.

Salads

Try adding the following to your salads so they have plenty of substance:

- black beans
- sliced boiled eggs
- garbanzo beans
- avocado slices
- Pace salsa (or any sugar free salsa)

The goal is to reach around 1,000 to 1,200 calories for the day, and since your breakfast and lunch together are only about 400, you can enjoy a significant dinner and feel full. Four oz. of meat is around 200 calories and vegetables are about 50 calories a cup for broccoli, green beans, and cauliflower. You will have to add calorie-dense ingredients to your salad to get to 1000 calories.

Salad Dressings

Because you are eliminating wheat, dairy, refined sugar, and bad oils from your diet, you will need to make your own salad dressings. Go to the recipes section in the back of this workbook and make your own delicious dressing.

Hormone Balance

Research the value of bioidentical progesterone cream. It is based on the research of Dr. John Lee who explains that balanced hormones, detoxing your body and eating whole healthy foods, all go together to accomplish health. For further, detailed information about hormone balance and the use of bioidentical progesterone cream read *Dr. Deanna's Healing Handbook.*

How to Use a Progesterone Cream

Men: 5 to 10 mg daily

Women: If you still have a menstrual cycle, use one 20 mg pump a day, on your stomach and inside of your arms, from day 12 to day 28 of your cycle.

I am past menopause, and so I skip the first five days of the calendar month, and use one pump at night for the rest of the month. Do not use any lotion on the skin where you are applying the progesterone cream. Most lotions contain mineral oils, parabens, sulfates, and phthalates, which are hormone disrupters and can block the absorption of progesterone. Progesterone is the precursor hormone--your body uses it to make estrogen, estrodiol, testosterone, thyroid hormone, etc. Use bioidentical—a progesterone that is identical to the progesterone your body makes naturally. It is an amazing aid in combating hot flashes, postpartum depression, and other hormone imbalance symptoms. In America, we are exposed to so much that disrupts our hormone balance. Even if you don't have hormone imbalance symptoms, you can use the progesterone cream for maintenance. When your hormones are balanced you will sleep better, notice clearer thinking and a positive life outlook.

As a single mom on a tight budget, it took some convincing to change my health for the better. Now I understand so much more about how to take care of my body, and help my children achieve a healthy lifestyle by avoiding the foods and chemicals that their generation is saturated with. I want to be "fit to serve!"

Shopping List

Bulk food list for Sam's Club/Costco

- Unrefined expeller pressed coconut oil
- Frozen mixed berries
- Frozen strawberries
- Frozen green beans
- Broccoli
- Red peppers
- Fresh organic spinach (Freeze ½ for shakes)
- Frozen California blend vegetables
- Cauliflower
- Shredded salad greens
- Granny Smith apples
- Avocados
- Quinoa
- Almond butter

Grocery store list

- Coconut milk in the can (look in Asian cooking section)
- Unsweetened almond milk
- Sweet potatoes
- Dijon mustard
- Pace brand salsa (or another that has no sugar)
- Stevia packets or the liquid which is sweeter and easier to mix (natural sugar substitute)

Healthy Snacks Ideas: protein bar, Granny Smith apple sliced and sprinkled with stevia and cinnamon, a cup of steamed green beans or broccoli, raw vegetables.

Protein Bar Recipe

- 2 cups vanilla protein powder
- 2 cups chocolate protein powder
- 1 can coconut milk
- 2 TB almond butter
- Dash of salt and a little extra stevia liquid if desired

Mix in large food processor or hand mix. Press into 9 X 13 pan. Cut into 20 squares. Each bar is approximately 75 calories each. Two bars and a Granny Smith apple can be used as a meal. If you prefer vanilla, use 4 cups vanilla protein, eliminate chocolate, and sprinkle the top with cinnamon.

Nutrition Tips

Your two shakes or one shake/one protein bar meal, will provide about 400 calories. You need 600-800 more calories through the day. You should never be hungry. Hungry will make you grumpy, tired, and less productive in your work and we can't have that! For snacks in between meals, make sure you stay under the additional 600-800 calories AND **avoid wheat, refined sugar, dairy and GMO oils like canola, corn, cottonseed, etc.** Remember, only protein kills your hunger, so a low fat protein snack is best. Here are some suggestions to make your eating more fun.

On your salad at dinner try adding a sliced, hard-boiled egg and ½ cup black beans. For a sweeter salad, throw on a few almonds with a half cup of sliced strawberries on top. I like adding ½ an avocado because it feels more like a creamy dressing without the bad fat. If you get hungrier in the morning, snack extra then; if at night, then save 150 calories for a bedtime snack.

To find out how many calories are in specific food, search online. After about a week, you will have learned many of the calorie amounts and won't have to do much research. Here are some foods I regularly eat, with their calorie values:

PROTEIN:	CALORIES:
Hard boiled egg	211
4 oz. chicken breast	140
4 oz. Cod	100

VEGGIES:	
½ cup white beans	150
½ cup pinto beans	118
½ cup black beans	115
1 cup sugar snap peas	70
1 cup broccoli	54
1 cup asparagus	40
1 cup green beans	34
1 cup zucchini	29
1 cup raw tomato	27
1 cup cauliflower	14
1 cup romaine lettuce	8
1 cup raw spinach	7

FRUIT:	
1 cup blueberries	83
1 Granny Smith apple	80
1 cup raspberries	64
1 cup strawberries	48

For making soup and casseroles:	
1 cup coconut milk	550
1 cup salsa	80
1 cup carrots	52
1 cup cabbage	40
1 cup unsweet almond milk	40
1 tsp. coconut oil	40

For added flavor sprinkle foods with stevia, cinnamon, nutmeg or pumpkin pie spice.

Food Journal - *What I ate today:*

_____

_____

_____

_____

_____

_____

_____

Comments - *How did I feel today & what did I learn?*

_____

_____

_____

_____

_____

_____

_____

What do I need to work on:

_____

_____

_____

_____

_____

_____

_____

_____

Day 2
The Order of Creation

We will begin our health transformation where God began—in the garden. God took chaos – Genesis 1:2, "And the earth was **without form, and void**; and darkness [was] upon the face of the deep - having no divine order, no life, and under a shroud of complete darkness." In Genesis, God created His garden as well as night and day, the heavens, water, dry land, grass, herb yielding seed, fruit tree yielding fruit after his kind, whose seed is in itself, sun, moon and stars, sea creatures, fowls that fly, cattle, creeping things, then man to whom God invested dominion over His creation.

God began His creation by setting a particular order, so that men and women formed of flesh and bone and in His own spiritual image, the crown of His creation, could live in abundant life. God first created the light and air, then dry land and water. Before creating life, he formed all things that were needed to give and support life. His creation began with order, and His divine order remains. When the earthly garden was prepared, God said,

> *Let the earth bring forth grass, the herb yielding seed, and the fruit tree yielding fruit after his kind, whose seed is in itself, upon the earth (v. 11).*

Then presenting sustenance to man,

> *…God said, Behold, I have given you every herb bearing seed, which is upon the face of all the earth, and every tree, in the which is the fruit of a tree yielding seed; to you it shall be for meat (v. 29).*

God's order in giving plants life, after light, air, earth, and water had been prepared, demonstrated the wisdom of the Creator and the naturalness of His working. The earth was ordered to contain all the elements; then God put in the life vessel to carry on His plan from generation to generation - seed.

John Calvin observes God's blessing to man and the rest of His creation to "be fruitful and multiply" according to the divine plan set down in the garden.

> *Nor was it meaningless that the words of benediction were addressed to the creatures; it was designed to teach that the force of the Divine word was not meant to be transient, but, being infused into their natures, to take root and constantly bear fruit.*

We will prayerfully consider in the weeks ahead what our responsibility to God is regarding the seed. God defined it as "herb yielding seed, yielding fruit after its kind, whose seed is in itself." What are the results of stepping outside of God's definition of seed, and eating from the "new and improved" modified and altered sterile food supply?

> *Give us this day, our daily bread. Matthew 6:11*

Bread is a staple food in every culture, and Jesus taught his disciples to pray for "daily bread." Similar prayers were prayed by the poorest man in scripture, Job, and the richest man in scripture, Solomon. Today we will learn why, when we pray for the most basic nourishment God gives, we must avoid the grains that are now damaging to our health. Here's why.

Health Lesson: No Wheat. What?

After eating the Standard American Diet all my life, it was hard for me to imagine what to eat without wheat! If you want to know everything there is to know about wheat and how it has been dramatically altered since the days of our grandparents, order a copy of Dr. William Davis's book, *Wheat Belly*. But if you are too busy to read a whole book, you can learn what you need to know by reading this article—"Why 80 percent of people worldwide will soon stop eating wheat." It is a very serious component to our current health woes particularly in the industrialized world. You can find the article at multiple sites using your search engine.

Author Natasha Longo explains the many health risks associated with the consumption of wheat which are more numerous than the nutritional benefits claimed by the wheat industry. According to Longo, there is an association between grain consumption and the following: neurological impairment, dementia, heart disease, cataracts, diabetes, arthritis and visceral fat accumulation, gluten intolerances and bloating. Approximately 700 million tons of wheat are now cultivated worldwide making it the second most-produced grain after corn.

The majority of wheat is processed into 60% extraction, bleached white flour. Sixty percent extraction–the standard for most wheat products means that 40% of the original wheat grain is removed. Not only do we have an unhealthy, modified, and hybridized strain of wheat, we also remove and further degrade its nutritional value by processing it.

Unfortunately, 40 percent of what is removed includes the bran and the germ of the wheat grain–its most nutrient-rich parts. In the process of making 60 percent extraction flour, over half of the vitamin B1, B2, B3, E, folic acid, calcium, phosphorus, zinc, copper, iron, and fiber are lost.

Any processed foods with wheat are akin to poison for the body since they cause more health risks than benefits. The body does not recognize processed wheat as food. Nutrient absorption from processed wheat products is thus inconsequential with almost no nutritional value.

Whole wheat products are based on modern wheat strains created by irradiation of wheat seeds and embryos with chemicals, gamma rays, and high-dose X-rays to induce mutations. Whether you consume 10% or 100% of wheat is irrelevant, since you're still consuming a health damaging grain that will not benefit, advance or even maintain your health in any way.

"In my practice of over two decades, we have documented that for every ten people with digestive problems, obesity, irritable bowel syndrome, diabetes, arthritis and even heart disease, eight out of ten have a problem with wheat. Once we remove wheat from their diets, most of their symptoms disappear within three to six months." -- Dr. Marcia Alvarez

Author of *Wheat Belly* and preventive cardiologist William Davis, MD, says wheat's new biochemical code causes hormone disruption that is linked to diabetes and obesity. "It is not my contention that it is in everyone's best interest to cut back on wheat; it is my belief that *complete elimination* is in everyone's best health interests," says Dr. Davis. "In my view, that's how bad this thing called 'wheat' has become."

We recommend that you look at the research available on the new hybridized wheat, and make a commitment to eliminate all grains from your diet during our transition to health.

WHAT TO DO:

Compare the Healthy Living Cheat Sheet to what is in your pantry. Purchase some brown rice and quinoa which will be our healthy wheat substitutes for the next 30 days. You will be amazed at how much better your wheat-free body functions!

Healthy Living Cheat sheet

HOW TO FILL YOUR PLATE:

Green Veggies
1/2 of your plate
Kale, Chard, Mustard Greens, Spinach, Broccoli,
Asparagus

Lean Protein
1/4 of your plate
Free-range turkey, fresh wild fish, free-range
chicken, grass-fed beef once per week

Good Carbs
1/8 your plate
Brown Rice, Quinoa, Sweet Potatoes, Beets, Carrots

Good Fat
1/8 of your plate
Nut Oils, Olive Oils, Salmon, Avocado, Flax

HOW TO MAKE A MEAL REPLACEMENT SHAKE:
2 scoops of pea protein powder
1/2 to 1 scoop fiber supplement
Ice (optional)
1/4 to 1/2 cup berries (optional)

Mix with your choice of the following liquids:
8 oz. cold water
8 oz. unsweetened almond, flax or coconut milk

Add one serving of healthy fat (optional):
1 tsp coconut oil, flax seeds, avocado, almonds or almond
butter.

HOW TO MAKE A RECOVERY SHAKE:
(Drink within 30 min. of a 60+ min. workout)
1-2 scoops of pea protein powder
1/4 cup refrigerated, unsweetened almond milk
1/4 cup frozen berries or a good carb
1/2 banana or 1/2 cup pineapple
Water/Ice for consistency

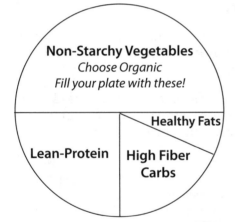

Non-Starchy Vegetables
Choose Organic
Fill your plate with these!

Healthy Fats

Lean-Protein

High Fiber Carbs

> **REPLACE 1-2 MEALS PER DAY WITH VEGAN PROTEIN SHAKES TO SATISFY HUNGER AND BOOST ENERGY!**

ELIMINATE

- Dairy
- Gluten
- Soy
- Peanuts & Peanut Butter
- Sugar, Honey, Maple Syrup
- Artificial Sweeteners
- Coffee

- Alcohol
- ALL FRUIT EXCEPT: berries, green apples, lemons & limes
- Pork
- Farm-Raised Fish
- Non Cage-Free Eggs
- Non Free-Range Chicken

- All Beef, other than grass fed
- White Potatoes
- Corn
- Nitrates
- MSG
- Vinegar

Food Journal - *What I ate today:*

_____

_____

_____

_____

_____

_____

_____

Comments - *How did I feel today & what did I learn?*

_____

_____

_____

_____

_____

_____

_____

What do I need to work on:

_____

_____

_____

_____

_____

_____

_____

Day 3

The Danger of Providing for the Flesh

But put ye on the Lord Jesus Christ, and make not provision for the flesh, to fulfil the lusts thereof. Romans 13:14

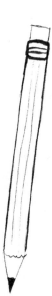

Those with more than a utilitarian view of food can fall prey to appetites. Are you spending an inordinate amount of time each day making provision for the "flesh," that is, thinking about and preparing foods? Even when we are not hungry – we eat.

We tend, in these days of extraordinary plenty, to plan events around food more than people and eat for entertainment. We have come a long way since the days when most, if not all, families had a connection to growing their own foods on farms and/or smaller kitchen gardens. Many have now lost sight of the original and true nature of food and what constitutes fuel for the body. This verse gives us counsel in breaking the focus of life that is unnaturally fixed on eating - appetites. Let us put on the Lord Jesus Christ. May our desires turn to Him more intensely than misplaced thoughts toward gaining comfort and pleasure from food.

Today we are going to look at ways those desires are manipulated by food additives, and even food addictions. By understanding what has happened to the food system, we can be equipped to find and eat clean and pure food, as we make no provision for the flesh. Our appetites are too often manipulated today. Let us be wise and aware, so as not to be driven by a fleshly sense of taste. Let us seek foods to fuel our bodies for health and service in the Kingdom!

Health Lesson:

GLOSSARY OF CLEAN EATING

Today we will look more closely at the food in our kitchens, and eliminate four genetically modified foods. Here are some suggestions to think about:

1. **WHOLE FOODS** (aka God foods) - they grow on trees or from the ground. Ask yourself, "was this food ALIVE?"

2. **PROCESSED FOOD** (aka man food) - they contain loads of additives, preservatives, artificial flavors/sweeteners/colors (think chemicals).

3. **ORGANIC** - free of pesticides/herbicides (look for a round green/white USDA Organic label on the front of all foods). Organic fruits/veggies contain 40% more antioxidant vitamins than their conventionally grown counterparts.

4. **Non-GMO** - GMO stands for Genetically Modified Organism. This means man took a whole food into the lab, and cross bred or altered its DNA in a Petri dish, so it can be doused with a broad spectrum plant killer such as Roundup, and not die. The Roundup is in the soil, absorbed into our food, and damages the gut flora that are responsible for 80 percent of our immune system. Eliminate all non-organic soy, corn, sugar, and canola/cottonseed oils. These are the "Big 4" that are in more than 70 percent of the food in the grocery store.

5. **FREE-RANGE, CAGE FREE & GRASS-FED meats/eggs** - "Free range" applies to poultry your chicken/turkey was allowed to roam as it was intended in open space (not confined). ⌐ for "cage-free" eggs as this means your egg-laying hen was also free-range and vegetarian fed. "Grass fed and finished" applies to your beef. This ensures your cattle were fed as it was also intended - allowed to roam freely and eat on the pasture. Most US cattle, as well as farm-raised fish, are fed a GMO corn diet to fatten them up and you are getting a high fat, high chemical result. All conventional meats are LOADED with added hormones and antibiotics.

WHAT TO DO:

Remove the four major GMO products from your pantry—Corn, soy, sugar, and canola/cottonseed oil. (Includes High Fructose Corn Syrup and Soy Lecithin)

Go to multimedia section of the www.AppetiteforGod.com website to watch a short video that explains how GM food affects the bacteria in your gut. The video is entitled, "GMO."

Also in the multimedia section, read "The Extraordinary Science of Addictive Junk Food" from the New York Times Magazine; then use the discussion questions to respond to the article as a group:

Questions for Group Discussion:

1. Michael Moss, investigative reporter for the New York Times, asserts that food addiction is a deliberate goal of America's largest food companies: Kraft, Nabisco, General Mills, Proctor & Gamble, Coca-Cola, and Mars. Do you think companies should have the right to process food to create more hunger?

2. Why do companies put flavor enhancers in our food?

3. One fourth to one third of adults are obese. Do food processing companies have any responsibility for the obesity epidemic? What do you think they should do?

4. According to Moss, "there is a conscious effort on behalf of food manufacturers to get you hooked on foods that are convenient and inexpensive." People spend $1 trillion annually on processed foods. Why?

5. Should we choose foods for their bliss point, mouth feel, or craving? Why is this a problem?

6. How does sugar compare to cocaine?

7. What is the problem with processed meats (bacon, sausage, lunch meat, etc.)?

8. How can you diminish your craving for junk food?

BEEF
Grass Fed vs Grain Fed

Cattle eat their natural diet of grasses.

No antibiotics.

No hormones.

Cattle roam in an open pasture to feed.

Cattle naturally take 1.5-2 years to mature.

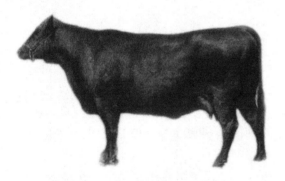

Most beef sold in stores & restaurants.

Cattle eat 90% corn, 10% other:
Such as forage & cheap high-energy feeds like candy, starch, bakery waste, potato waste, pasta, chicken litter and meat processing waste.

+Antibiotics
29 million pounds on American livestock in 2009 for illnesses and growth promotion.

+Hormones
Implants or injections are used to increase growth rate by 10-15%.

Confined Feedlots
Restricting movement prevents cattle from using energy so that they fatten more quickly.

1 Year to Maturity
The combination of high-energy foods, drugs and confinement turns cows into cheap meat in half the time.

Meat composition of grass fed cows is significantly healthier when analyzed for fat and nutrient content:

- 2-4x more Omega 3
- 5x more CLA*
- More vitamins & minerals

4x MORE FAT
per 3 oz. serving

*CLA is a healthy fat that has been linked to a reduced risk of cancer.

Information by mcmichaelchiro.com, Used by Permission

16

Food Journal - *What I ate today:*

_____

_____

_____

_____

_____

_____

_____

Comments - *How did I feel today & what did I learn?*

_____

_____

_____

_____

_____

_____

_____

What do I need to work on:

_____

_____

_____

_____

_____

_____

_____

Day 4

Choosing Food For Health

Prove thy servants, I beseech thee, ten days; and let them give us pulse to eat, and water to drink. Then let our countenances be looked upon before thee, and the countenance of the children that eat of the portion of the king's meat: and as thou seest, deal with thy servants. So he consented to them in this matter, and proved them ten days. And at the end of ten days their countenances appeared fairer and fatter in flesh than all the children which did eat the portion of the king's meat. Daniel 1: 12-15

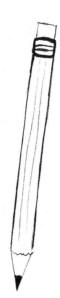

The Book of Daniel begins in a time of Judah being forcibly carried off to a foreign land and government. The Babylonian government surveyed the captive population and cut out a young leadership class to be indoctrinated in all their ways, language, customs, religion, etc., to likely aid in assimilating the foreign captive population into the kingdom, a very practical method for keeping the peace.

Daniel's first personal and religious challenge from the foreign government had to do with food. I have often read Daniel and focused on Daniel's faithfulness, but thinking now from the Babylonian perspective, today it doesn't seem too strange a business that food restrictions would figure into the government's grooming of young foreigners for leadership.

Sure there are dietary laws the Jews followed – meat preparation was particularly regulated – and no doubt the Babylonian method of meat preparation would be unacceptable to a practicing Jew like Daniel, but let's consider why transformation of the captives should begin with food.

Babylon provisioned their best foods upon the young captives and it should come as no surprise that the US government today has a recommended food system that is intended for safety and keeping quality high. The US food system is obviously corrupted by more than GMOs as evidenced by the fact many are sick and many are obese, feeding the growing rates of chronic illnesses instead of the people.

America is not thriving despite the government's regulation of food production and safety, the guidance of food pyramids, subsidies to farmers, industrialized farming which depletes the soil and provides less and less nutrition, and the sanction and operation of a food system designed to deliver out-of-season foods year round via worldwide transport.

Daniel bargained with his handlers – the government regulators - to be allowed to narrow his palate to consume a fare of pulse (pulses are: dry beans like pinto beans, kidney beans navy beans, dry peas, lentils and others) and water – a lowly food grown from the land – but carrying the essentials for good health and keeping peace with God. The lesson is not just about beans and peas, but that governments are not the final authority, and as Daniel found early on in a foreign land, they can't be blindly trusted to deliver good food for the body or the soul. It is up to us, like Daniel, to take control of our food sources and not blindly follow what for many isn't working to bring health to our families and nation.

Health Lesson:

WHY do I want to eat organic? Does it REALLY make THAT much of a difference? But doesn't it cost more? How can I tell what's organic in the grocery?

Why? Because organic foods are non-toxic and unaltered with no pesticides, herbicides, GMOs, they are nutritionally sound and give your body the fuel it needs. Take a peek at the nutrient comparison between organic and conventional. Mind-blowing, huh?

Cost? Yes, organic costs more. It's a supply-demand thing and until the population demands otherwise, organic will be the underdog and take more resources to create/transport. Buy organic as much as your budget allows.

Can't do it all organic? Consider the items on your "Dirty Dozen & Clean 15" list below. The Dirty Dozen are your dirtiest fruits/veggies (most pesticides, etc). You absolutely want to buy these organic because of the amount of chemicals used to treat them or the nature of their thin skin or absorbency. Your Clean 15 list, on the other hand, uses little/no chemicals and/or have thick skin that is not permeated by chemical exposure. So it's okay to buy these conventional.

How do you spot the difference?

Usually, it's pretty easy, look for labeling on the shelves, the USDA organic logo and the actual sticker on the produce. Conventional produce will have a 4-digit number starting with 4. Organic produce will have a 5-digit number starting with 9. Here's a quick tip on your apples: If it's pretty and shiny...it's DIRTY! That shine is actually a chemical wax. Apples top the Dirty Dozen list, so skip the shine and go organic!

WHAT TO DO:

Go to your local grocery store and browse the organic section, or visit Trader Joes and Whole Foods, but even those stores will have plenty of processed food to avoid. Find items you like and that fit your budget. For me, the "Simple Truth" brand at my local Kroger is great. I get organic green beans and broccoli at Costco for less money than the non-organics at the grocery. The organic salad makings are only a few cents more than the others, and they are pesticide free!

Dirty Dozen

Buy Organic:

Apples	Peaches*
Bell Peppers	Potatoes*
Blueberries (domestic)	Spinach
Celery	Strawberries
Cucumbers	
Grapes*	**+PLUS**
Lettuce	Green Beans
Nectarines* (imported)	Kale/Greens

+PLUS
Green Beans
Kale/Greens
Pesticide residues of special conern.

*Not recommend during this 40 day program

Clean Fifteen

Lowest in Pesticides:

Asparagus	Mangoes*
Avocado	Mushrooms
Cabbage	Onions
Cantaloupe (domestic)	Pineapples*
Corn*	Sweet Peas
Eggplant	Sweet Potatoes
Grapefruit	Watermelon*
Kiwi	

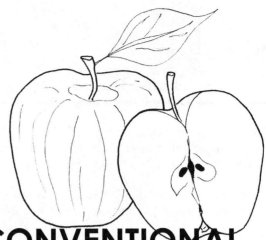

ORGANIC VS. CONVENTIONAL

Minerals (in milliequivalents)							
Vegetables Type of Soil Management	Calcium	Magnesium	Potassium	Sodium	Magnanese	Iron	Copper
Snap Beans							
Organic	40.5	60.0	99.7	8.6	60.0	227.0	69.0
Conventional	15.5	14.8	29.1	0.0	2.0	10.0	3.0
Cabbage							
Organic	60.0	43.6	148.3	20.4	13.0	94.0	48.0
Conventional	17.5	15.6	53.7	0.8	2.0	20.0	0.4
Lettuce							
Organic	71.0	49.3	176.5	12.2	169.0	516.0	60.0
Conventional	16.0	13.1	53.7	0.0	1.0	1.0	3.0
Tomatoes							
Organic	23.0	59.2	148.3	6.5	68.0	1938.0	53.0
Conventional	4.5	4.5	58.6	0.0	1.0	1.0	0.0
Spinach							
Organic	96.0	293.9	257.0	69.5	117.0	1584.0	0.0
Conventional	47.5	46.9	84.0	0.8	1.0	19.0	0.5

Research conducted by Firman E. Bear at Rutgers University in the Natural Gardener's Catalog (1995)

A Word About Coffee — Coffee is the most heavily sprayed food crop in the world. If you do not eliminate coffee from your diet all together, it is the ***most important item to buy organic***. The processing and pesticide use are only heavier on nonfood items such as cotton. Ask for organic coffee at your local coffee shop. Don't settle for anything else!

Food Journal - *What I ate today:*

_____
_____
_____
_____
_____
_____
_____

Comments - *How did I feel today & what did I learn?*

_____
_____
_____
_____
_____
_____
_____
_____
_____

What do I need to work on:

_____
_____
_____
_____
_____
_____
_____
_____

Day 5

Abundant life—what does it mean?

The thief cometh not, but for to steal, and to kill, and to destroy: I am come that they might have life, and that they might have it more abundantly. John 10:10

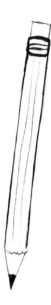

I remember a Christmas vacation that ended badly. I returned to my home after a week out of town with family to find that my house had been robbed and cleaned out to the bare walls. It was shocking to think that someone came into MY house and took MY belongings and MY children's toys. A thief cares only for his own selfish ends. His life is wasted on hurting himself for elusive pleasure until his seared conscience no longer condemns his wrongdoing.

Food whose only purpose is to addict the eater and provide a profit for the processor is a thief. Salt, fat, sugar, and chemically enhanced foods rob us of long life, productive life, fulfilling life. It brings chronic suffering through heart disease, diabetes, and dementia. Make no mistake—it will eventually kill and destroy. This is not abundant life.

The Good Shepherd gives pasture to His sheep. He makes a way for them to have real food that will secure the health needed to go in and out of the demands of life. Abundant life is full of strength, beauty, growth, and reproduction, and is strongly resistant to disease.

Will you throw the thief out of your household? Will you be a witness to others of the abundant life that we have because our God cares for us? The children of Israel were admired by nations around them for their exceptional health. They surrendered their appetites to God. Will you? We are still called to abundant life here and hereafter.

Health Lesson:

Scientific American published an article in 2011 titled "Dirt Poor" which explains how soil depletion has made our food less nutritious. They report,

Modern intensive agricultural methods have stripped increasing amounts of nutrients from the soil in which the food we eat grows. Sadly, each successive generation of fast-growing, pest-resistant carrot is truly less good for you than the one before.

Scientific American cites a study published in the *Journal of the American College of Nutrition* that studied U.S. Department of Agriculture nutritional data from 1950 and 1999 for 43 different vegetables and fruits, identifying declines in the amount of protein, calcium, phosphorus, iron, riboflavin, and vitamin C. The study concludes, "Efforts to breed new varieties of crops that provide greater yield, pest resistance and climate adaptability have allowed crops to grow bigger and more rapidly, but their ability to manufacture or uptake nutrients has not kept pace with their rapid growth."

Foods that are certified organic are GMO free. When I shop, I remember the four big offenders—**corn, soy, sugar, and oil.** I limit my oil intake to coconut oil, avocados, olive and walnut oil. These are healthy oils, and replace harmful GMO and saturated fats that are more difficult to digest. When you eliminate sugar and high fructose corn syrup, you have skipped every inside grocery aisle! Your choices become small servings of organic grass fed beef and poultry, wild caught cold-water fish, and fresh or frozen organic fruits and vegetables. Thankfully eating a more clean and natural diet is not only disease preventive it is cost effective and affordable. It is time to abandon chemically treated and altered pseudo-food and re-discover the real nutrition that fuels our minds and bodies.

For a full discussion of the shift from organic gardening to agribusiness monoculture, see Chapter 1 of *Dr. Deanna's Healing Handbook*. Learn the principles of health, and you won't be tempted to eat junk.

WHAT TO DO:

On this "AVOID LIST'" everything is either allergenic, addictive or acidic. You can do this!!! Buy a few staples from the "include" list like stevia, almonds, cage-free eggs, and a few avocados that will have to sit a few days to soften and be ready to eat!

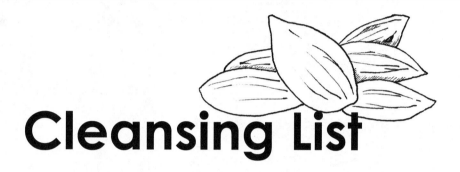

Cleansing List

ELIMINATE:

- Alcohol
- Artificial sweeteners
- Beef that is not grassfed
- Coffee
- Corn
- Dairy
- Non cage-free eggs
- Farm-raised fish
- All fruit EXCEPT limes, lemons, green apples & berries
- Gluten
- Nitrates
- MSG
- Peanuts & peanut butter
- Pork
- Soy
- Sugar, honey & maple syrup
- Vinegar
- White potatoes

INCLUDE:

- Almond, coconut & flax milk
- Almond butter
- Almonds (raw), walnuts & pecans
- Avocado
- Beef, grassfed (1x per week)
- Brown rice
- Chicken and turkey, free-range
- Coconut sugar
- Eggs, cage-free
- Green & herb teas
- Legumes
- Non starchy vegetables
- Organic green apples & berries
- Olive, avocado, coconut & walnut oil
- Quinoa
- Stevia or Xylitol
- Sweet potatoes, yams & turnips
- Wild-caught, cold water fish (1x per week)

Food Journal - *What I ate today:*

_____

_____

_____

_____

_____

_____

_____

_____

Comments - *How did I feel today & what did I learn?*

_____

_____

_____

_____

_____

_____

_____

_____

What do I need to work on:

_____

_____

_____

_____

_____

_____

_____

DAY 6

Hezekiah was supposed to pass it on

But Hezekiah rendered not again according to the benefit done unto him; for his heart was lifted up: therefore there was wrath upon him, and upon Judah and Jerusalem. II Chronicles 32:25

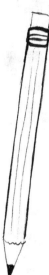

Hezekiah was a great reformer and king, and at the peak of his life, he lost his health. He prayed to God, who added fifteen years to his life. What did God expect from Hezekiah during those 15 years? He was given a great gift—the gift of health, and in this verse, we learn that God expected him to use that benefit to help others. Instead he became proud—"his heart was lifted up."

Be careful as you learn during these forty days. God will give you the gift of renewed health as you have set aside this time to seek Him and obey His prompting. But don't use your newfound understanding to beat others over the head. Be patient. Your loved ones will want to know after you have walked the new walk for a few months. If we become arrogant as Hezekiah did, everyone around us suffers.

Have a humble spirit as you go to God with your needs, and God will give you the opportunity to pass on your benefit to others. Our family has been living this healthy lifestyle for two years, and I am so thankful He has allowed me to tell you my story. Like Hezekiah, my life has been lengthened, and my family is enjoying God's gift. I want to keep my heart right, so the whole nation around me is blessed with supernatural health.

Health Lesson:

There is a huge variation in quality and nourishment found in protein supplements, and it is essential to your success to choose a protein supplement that satisfies your hunger and tastes good. I use a protein supplement that combines yellow pea, cranberry and rice proteins, and is fortified with extra vitamins and minerals. It mixes with water for a complete amino acid profile (providing all 20 essential amino acids your body needs), and actually tastes good - mixed with water with nothing added!

Using a protein supplement was key for my daughter and me to transition from the SAD (Standard American Diet) way of eating to a permanent healthy lifestyle. Avoid whey protein which is dairy based. The National Institute of Diabetes and Digestive and Kidney Diseases estimates that 30 to 50 million Americans are lactose intolerant. Lactose is the sugar in dairy; casein is the protein. Casein can become an allergy irritant. Dairy products are the leading cause of food allergy, although many may not recognize it as the source of diarrhea, constipation and fatigue, or frequent sinus/ear infections or even asthma. You may not have recognizable symptoms from digesting dairy, but it could still cause systemic inflammation, which may result in chronic mucous production. Studies point to a correlation between whey and diabetes, because it breaks down so quickly and may overstress the body's insulin producing mechanisms at the cellular level.

We also recommend that you avoid soy protein because of its endocrine disrupting properties. Make sure your protein is not heated in the extraction process, and delivers all of your body's needs for essential amino acids.

WHAT TO DO:

Most people already have a blender, but if not, think about buying a single serving blender. They come with six individual cups, and will greatly reduce your kitchen time. I have used the GE, Bella, and Magic Bullet. I like the GE the best, but any of them with 16 to 20 oz. cups are good. They are available at Department Stores for under $20, or the Magic Bullet for around $50.

Check out the strawberries, blueberries, blackberries and raspberries at your local Sam's Club or Costco where you can get a 3 pound bag of organic berries for under $10. Whole Foods often has great prices on berries as well. Put a few pounds of frozen berries in your freezer to blend in shakes. A pound of fresh organic spinach or kale can be frozen to add to the shakes as well.

You can use unsweetened almond milk, add a handful of spinach, or other greens in a chocolate shake and it's delicious. If weight loss is your goal, stick to the basic shake recipe. There is no reason to add "milk" of any sort and especially not cow's milk. If you are at optimal weight and want improved health, you can add things like almond butter, frozen cherries, or more berries for variety. More shake recipes are available on www.AppetiteforGod.com. **Don't add any extras during this program.** Small additions make a huge difference in the amount of weight loss.

The Basic Protein Shake:

- 2 scoops protein powder
- ½ cup frozen berries (add ice if using fresh)
- 9 oz filtered water
- 1 scoop of fiber to morning shake
- Blend and go!

Food Journal - *What I ate today:*

_____

_____

_____

_____

_____

_____

_____

Comments - *How did I feel today & what did I learn?*

_____

_____

_____

_____

_____

_____

_____

_____

_____

What do I need to work on:

_____

_____

_____

_____

_____

_____

_____

Day 7

Standing Alone in the Right Place

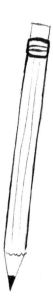

All things are lawful for me, but I will not be brought under the power of any. I Corinthians 6:12

One of the greatest obstacles to getting healthy is the sense of social isolation that can result when we stop eating the SAD or Standard American Diet everyone else is eating. Because the consequences of toxic foods don't appear in a 24-hour window, people can't see the need to give up sugar and processed foods. They do not know they are addicted. I know I certainly was. It is really pretty silly to think that if food doesn't make you sick today, it can't be bad for you. So the easy path is chosen for fast, easy, tasty foods and many people come under the power of their food addictions.

A few people do seem to get away with bad eating for 50 years, but one never knows about the quality of their physical lives. I made a physical and spiritual decision that I would not be under the power of food cravings. I decided to take control of my health future and to break my strong addiction to unhealthy foods. I wanted to do my part to secure energy and health to be ready for whatever God had for me to do in His kingdom. Are you under the power of sugar? Chocolate? Ice cream? Bread? Fast food? It is time to break that stronghold and not just for your physical health but also for your spiritual health!

Health Lesson:

Dr. William Davis recommends that we leave grains alone. Wheat, rice flour, tapioca, and potato starch spike the blood sugar, and overburden your pancreas, kidneys, and liver. High blood sugar is associated with cardiovascular disease, cataracts, hypertension, atherosclerosis, and arthritis. Fifty percent of all calories consumed world-wide come from grains. According to Dr. Davis, it's a sure prescription for an epidemic of diabetes and metabolic syndrome.

Dr. Mercola has published an article on the health benefits of fiber. He says, "Whole grains are not the best source of fiber as they contain anti-nutrients and glutinous "binding" proteins. Vegetables, nuts and seeds are the most healthful sources of fiber."

If you think of psyllium seeds that turn water into Jell-O and gag you going down, that is not what I am talking about when I say fiber.

Fiber should be completely soluble—some of my clients actually put it in their coffee! It should dissolve in your morning shake and keep you fuller longer. Fiber is well known for its benefit in keeping the colon "moving," but it does much more. The Mayo Clinic recommends fiber to lower your risk of diabetes and heart disease. Fiber lowers blood cholesterol levels, can reduce blood pressure and inflammation, and aids in weight loss. Since our goal in this 40 Days is total overall health improvement, adding fiber to our program is an essential contribution to reaching our goals. He names nine specific health conditions that may benefit from increased fiber intake: blood sugar control, heart health, stroke, weight loss, skin health, diverticulitis, hemorrhoids, irritable bowel syndrome, gallstones and kidney stones.

The rest of Dr. Mercola's article "The Health Benefits of Fiber" is available in the multimedia section at www.AppetitforGod.com.

WHAT TO DO:

Enjoy a salad of fresh greens and vegetables today. As you have already found out, all those bottles of salad dressings are full of sugar, chemical preservatives and genetically modified oils (canola and cottonseed). For 30 days, we will use delicious fresh fat free dressings that you can make in your mini-blender. Choose one of the salad dressing recipes in the back of the book that resembles the old junk dressing you thought tasted good, and blend it up. You will save calories, and retrain your taste buds to avoid the addictive false foods that have negatively impacted your health.

Throughout this workbook, we will avoid wheat and the four main GMO's—corn, soy, sugar, and canola/cottonseed oil. Dr. William Davis reports that his patients who went on a wheat-free diet for three months reported that acid reflux disappeared and the cyclic cramping and diarrhea of irritable bowel syndrome were gone, energy improved, sleep was deeper, and rashes disappeared which had been present for many years. Also rheumatoid arthritis pain improved or disappeared, and asthma symptoms improved or resolved. Athletes reported better performance.

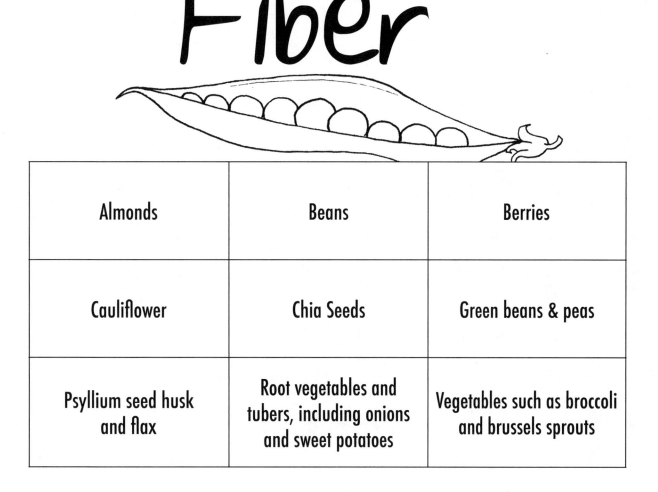

Fiber

Almonds	Beans	Berries
Cauliflower	Chia Seeds	Green beans & peas
Psyllium seed husk and flax	Root vegetables and tubers, including onions and sweet potatoes	Vegetables such as broccoli and brussels sprouts

Food Journal - *What I ate today:*

_____
_____
_____
_____
_____
_____
_____

Comments - *How did I feel today & what did I learn?*

_____
_____
_____
_____
_____
_____
_____

What do I need to work on:

_____
_____
_____
_____
_____
_____

DAY 8

A Prayer for Help

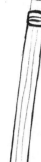

If any of you lack wisdom, let him ask of God, that giveth to all men liberally, and upbraideth not; and it shall be given him. James 1:5

Dear God, I have been unwise in my food decisions. It is discouraging to learn so many new things about the food I have eaten all of my life, and realize I have fallen into the traps of advertising and convenience that have hurt my health. You have commanded me, "be not deceived," so I will face the truth, and I will learn with courage to act. And as James instructed, I am asking for Your wisdom to make the changes in my life that will make me fit for service, and protect my family from mental and physical instability. Thank you God for being the generous Giver. I will respond with holy patience, not condemning myself or others, but receiving with gratitude the precious gift of right knowledge that leads to life. ***"Show me thy ways, Oh Lord; teach me thy paths"*** Psalm 25:4. In Jesus' name I pray.

Health Lesson: No fear of fat!

I've been reading Dr. Perlmutter's book, *The Better Brain* today. Your brain needs fat. I am taking Omega-3's daily, but there is so much more to keeping your mind healthy and sharp. Here are excerpts from an article he has written that gives you the quick summary on fat and ways to solve our bad fat problems. I recommend his books!

The Secrets of Healthy Fats

As a culture, we've been conditioned to believe that low-fat foods are healthy. "This is not predicated on any science," says David Perlmutter, MD, author of the upcoming book, *Grain Brain: The Surprising Truth about Wheat, Carbs, and Sugar¬—Your Brain's Silent Killers.*

In low-fat processed foods, he points out, the fat has been replaced with carbohydrates, which increases our carbohydrate intake beyond our needs and causes blood-sugar spikes. This leads to a condition known as metabolic syndrome, which provokes belly fat, diabetes, and heart disease. Eating fat that is naturally present in foods is a critical part of the solution.

For example, conventional wisdom says that egg whites are healthier than whole eggs, but this isn't true. Scientists at the University of Connecticut, Storrs, compared the effects of whole eggs and a yolk-free egg substitute in a group of 40 men and women. For 12 weeks, they all followed a diet with no more than 30 percent of daily calories from carbohydrates (less than the American average), but half of them ate 3 eggs for breakfast while the others ate egg substitute. At the end of the trial, those who ate whole eggs had significantly lower levels of inflammatory cholesterol and better function of blood sugar and insulin.

The body needs a balance of two types of essential fats: anti-inflammatory omega-3s and pro-inflammatory omega-6s. In the days of caveman, it's estimated that the ratio of omega-6s to omega-3s was 2:1 or 1:1. In the modern American diet, that ratio is more like 20:1, which is highly pro-inflammatory and leads to diabetes, arthritis, heart disease, cancer, and weight gain. Several culprits contribute to this imbalance:

Problem - Inflammatory oils: Vegetable oils, such as canola and corn oils, are erroneously considered healthy options for cooking, and are abundant in processed and fast foods. Unfortunately, they're loaded with pro-inflammatory omega-6 fats.

Solution: Avoid processed and fast foods. Cook with healthy oils that withstand high heat, such as coconut, red palm, and rice bran oils. To dress salads, use extra virgin olive oil or flax seed oil. Add these after cooking, to preserve their beneficial fats.

Problem - Inflammatory meats: Commercial animal feed is made mostly from corn, rather than the grasses animals eat in natural habitats, and this alters the fat composition of meat. Rather than containing a healthy balance of essential fats, conventionally raised meat contains an inflated level of omega-6s.

Solution: Eat only grass-fed meats.

Problem - Inflammatory fish: Salmon, the richest source of omega-3 fats, is most often farm-raised (Atlantic Salmon). On conventional fish farms, salmon are fed corn, which raises their levels of inflammatory omega-6 fats. And high-heat cooking destroys omega-3 fats.

Solution: Eat wild salmon and other fish that are high in omega-3 fats. And cook your fish on low heat—preferably by poaching or steaming.

Problem - Inflammatory carbohydrates: Too many grains and too much sugar raise levels of chronic inflammation, increasing our need for anti-inflammatory omega-3 fats, which are already lacking in our diets.

Solution: Replace grains and sugar in your diet with non-starchy, above-ground vegetables; occasional fruit, such as apples or berries; and healthy plant sources of omega-3s, such as chia or flax seeds.

Different Types of Omega-3

"Increasing your omega-3 intake is probably the simplest thing you can do to improve your health," says Tom Gilhooly, MD, founder of The Centre for Nutritional Studies in Glasgow, Scotland. "Omega 3 fats have been the subject of more than 20,000 research papers," he says. Benefits include reduced risk of premature labor, less incidence of depression and ADHD, fewer PMS symptoms, and relief from inflammatory diseases.

Sources of Healthy Fats

A combination of supplements, oils, and seeds can restore the balance of fats in your diet. Many of these ingredients are found in nutritional powders, bars, and other food products.

Fish oil or a combination of EPA and DHA from algae or krill: Get 1–3 grams of a combination of EPA and DHA daily—quantities are listed on labels.

ALA: 1–2 grams daily. (One ounce of walnuts contains about 2.5 grams.) Flax seed oil contains the most available concentrated source of ALA

Coconut oil: Rich in a type of healthy saturated fat (see above), coconut oil also kills harmful bacteria in the gut.

Seeds: Chia and flax seeds are rich in omega-3 fats as well as other nutrients and fiber. Hemp seeds, also called hemp nuts, contain a combination of omega-3s and other healthy fats.

Extra virgin olive oil: High in healthy omega-9 fats, it's rich in antioxidants and is proven to enhance heart health. Drizzle it on food after cooking, or use it as a base for salad dressings. Dr. Perricone says Spanish Olive Oil is the best.

WHAT TO DO:

- Purge the kitchen & pantry of anything NON-nutrition focused. REMOVE TEMPTATION!

- Go grocery shopping. Use the Getting Started 4 page booklet on pages 5-8. Choose at least 10 items from the Nultrition Tips page so that you are set up for success.

- Set up your mini blender & shaker cup so that you have the right tools to start with!

- Pick up a food scale & tape measure if you don't have one. On page 154 you will find a chart for keeping a record of your weight and measurements, which begins on Day 11. Weigh at the same time each week in similar clothes (or no clothes!)

  - Watch a short video that explains the problem with sugar from *Dr. Deanna's Healing Handbook*. Go to multimedia section of the www.AppetiteforGod.com. The video is entitled, "Dangers of Sugar."

A Sample Day
with An Appetite for God

Wake Up
Cup of Detox Tea or Organic Coffee (if you need caffeine first thing)

Breakfast
Protein Shake with fiber supplement and probiotics.

Snack (optional)
Granny Smith apple sprinkled with stevia and cinnamon, protein bar, raw vegetables, small handful of nuts, seeds, or a tsp. of almond butter.

Lunch (4 hours after breakfast)
2 protein bars and a Granny Smith apple
- or -
A green salad topped with boiled eggs, black beans, vegetables and home made dressing.

Snack (optional)
See above

Dinner
A fist size of a lean protein, non-starchy veggies, a green salad topped with boiled eggs, black beans, vegetables and home made dressing. and a small amount of healthy fat.

DO NOT EAT AFTER 7PM!
Have a cup of detox tea if you get hungry.

Recovery Shake
If you work out intensely for an hour or more, make sure you have a recovery shake within 30 minutes of completing your workout. Your next meal will be within 4 hours when you become hungry. The recovery shake is in addition to your healthy meal plan.

Food Journal - *What I ate today:*

_____
_____
_____
_____
_____
_____
_____

Comments - *How did I feel today & what did I learn?*

_____
_____
_____
_____
_____
_____
_____
_____
_____

What do I need to work on:

_____
_____
_____
_____
_____
_____
_____
_____

DAY 9

The Mind of Christ: Caring for an Incredible Gift

But he that is spiritual judgeth all things, yet he himself is judged of no man. For who hath known the mind of the Lord, that he may instruct him? But we have the mind of Christ. I Corinthians 2:15-16

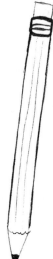

Paul makes an astonishing claim in his first letter to the Corinthians. He declares that spiritual people have the mind of Christ! At first I shrink back from embracing this truth, because it comes with such grave responsibility. But because it is true, I am compelled as a believer to make it true and act on it in my life.

Paul explains that those who have the mind of Christ are able to judge all things. Right judgment, or keenness of inquiry, the ability to analyze critically, and to discern pure truth are available to us who are spiritual. In chapter 5, Paul compares understanding the things of God to unleavened bread. A tiny sprinkling of yeast will cause the whole batch to rise. Our judgment is ruined by small encroachments of false influence. Our thought processes are also compromised by small amounts of toxic pseudo-foods.

If all one wants to understand is philosophy, the standards are much lower. You need only excellency of speech and wisdom (v. 1), enticing words (v. 4), and the wisdom of the world that is now abundant with a single keystroke.

But Jesus was no mere philosopher. He is a herald. He speaks and is Truth. We are quick to talk about Christianity as a change of the heart. But God also desires to quicken our minds so we can obey His command to remember, and respond with right judgment, spiritual transformation, and revelational understanding. The mind of Christ is not foggy or confused. It is characterized by clarity and comprehension.

In our program, we will learn ways to nourish the brain physiologically, which in turn enables us to respond fully to the Holy Spirit's daily teaching and revelation. Because we are given the mind of Christ, our obligation is great indeed to care for the mental faculties that would glorify His incredible gift.

Health Lesson:

Many people gain weight because they overeat from fast-food windows, in restaurants, and plan all of their social gatherings around food. Being healthy fits right in if you choose to hold the line. Have a protein shake before going to a party to curb your appetite, and lessen temptation. If you want to take a grain-free healthy dish to the family dinner, I recommend that you Google "Paleo Diet Recipes," or visit the website AgainstAllGrains.com.

Just for fun, Google an ingredient list of your favorite fast food. You will not be tempted to eat chicken nuggets or French fries again!

WHAT TO DO:

Organize your cupboards so you can make your shake in the morning, add fiber, probiotic digestive aid, and you're ready to start the day in less than 5 minutes!

Think about what your typical day will look like. A meal of protein shake. A meal of protein bars and a piece of fruit. A third meal of 4 oz. meat, and lots of fresh greens and vegetables. My daughter and I were amazed by our lack of hunger. The high protein content satisfies hunger! Drink at least 64 oz. of water daily to help support your detoxing organs as you release the toxins in the fat cells you are shedding.

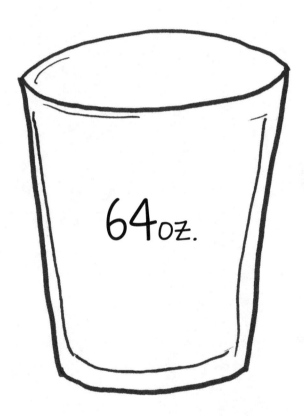

Food Journal - *What I ate today:*

_____
_____
_____
_____
_____
_____
_____
_____

Comments - *How did I feel today & what did I learn?*

_____
_____
_____
_____
_____
_____
_____
_____
_____

What do I need to work on:

_____
_____
_____
_____
_____
_____
_____
_____

Day 10

God's Gift of New Beginnings

Remember ye not the former things, neither consider the things of old. Behold, I will do a new thing; now it shall spring forth; shall ye not know it? I will even make a way in the wilderness, and rivers in the desert. The beast of the field shall honour me, the dragons and the owls: because I give waters in the wilderness, and rivers in the desert, to give drink to my people, my chosen. Isaiah 43:18-20

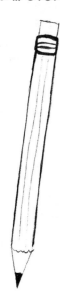

It is almost time to start putting into practice the many practical instructions we have studied that lead us from the Standard American Diet [SAD] to a healthful life of fitness in God's Kingdom. New beginnings can make you anxious, but there is also excitement as you consider you are partnering with God to be fit for service to Him. God gives us new beginnings. Isaiah and Jeremiah gave instruction to God's people at a very dark and discouraging time in their history. Many of us have been taken captive by changes in our food supply that have left us hungry and sick. God is offering you a new start, and He will make a way through this wilderness that isn't entirely clear to you just yet. He goes before us when we step out in faith to please Him. When the way seems hard, remember God, who brings rivers to the desert,is making a way for you. There is a breakthrough to freedom from food appetites that hinder your body and mind. We are His people, His chosen, and He is here. There is no looking back at the former things. Let's anticipate the new thing God is offering us, and run the race as servants who work at His pleasure.

Health Lesson:

Today I would like for us to consider the amazing healing properties of Vitamin D. *Dr. Deanna's Healing Handbook* explains the current research that connects the benefits of Vitamin D to reproductive health, shrinking uterine tumors, reducing risk of premenopausal breast cancer, improving bone and muscle health, and combating obesity. Vitamin D deficiency is linked to complications of pregnancy, multiple sclerosis, pneumonia, hypertension, and poor brain function. If you are concerned about chronic illness, you need to research the benefits of Vitamin D!

I began taking Vitamin D a few years ago when I found myself struggling with mild depression in the winter. Back then, it was labeled "Seasonal Affective Disorder," but I just called it getting the blues from living in Yucky Kentucky in February! If gray skies for weeks on end leave you feeling like you're not yourself, add 4,000 units of vitamin D to your health regimen.

Disclaimer: As always, we are not offering medical advice, and this suggestion is for educational purposes only.

WHAT TO DO:

The Getting Started Instructions are found in the first day of our workbook on pages 5-8. Using a highlighter, read through it again and highlight each item you need to buy before we start with our protein supplement weight loss/health/detox program. Make sure you have a can of coconut milk and almond butter to make a batch of protein bars tomorrow. If you only have vanilla protein powder, you can make the bars all vanilla, or make them all chocolate. I like vanilla bars with a tsp. of almond extract added, sprinkled on top with cinnamon. Planning ahead is critical every day for your success!

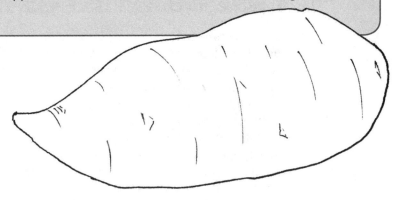

Watch a short video on "Being Normal." It's amazing how few people have a clue... Go to multimedia section of www.AppetiteforGod.com. The video is entitled, "Being Normal."

Food Journal - *What I ate today:*

_____
_____
_____
_____
_____
_____
_____
_____

Comments - *How did I feel today & what did I learn?*

_____
_____
_____
_____
_____
_____
_____
_____
_____

What do I need to work on:

_____
_____
_____
_____
_____
_____
_____
_____

DAY 11

Becoming Whole and Free

Jesus Christ maketh thee whole. Acts 9:34

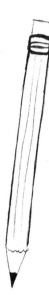

I have thought more in the last year about what it means to be whole than I have in my life. I have experienced a health transformation at a time in my life when most people are experiencing a health deterioration. I am dreaming of service to God in supernatural ways I could not possibly do if I were a prisoner to my food appetites as I was just a short time ago. Wholeness is breaking free. Wholeness is to stop the focus on fixing myself and pressing towards a high calling in Christ Jesus. (Philippians 3:14)

Though I am thrice widowed, I am NOT depressed or sick or lonely or needy or helpless or clueless. Jesus Christ makes me whole. I think Christians should stop asking, "How are you?" Instead let's ask, "How have you changed your world today?" This declaration of Peter needs to get under my skin—Jesus Christ makes me whole! It is glasses through which I see everything. Closely akin to Peter's statement is a declaration Jesus made to spiritually blind Pharisees, "If the Son therefore shall make you free, ye shall be free indeed."

I am struggling to define a life of wholeness and freedom. But I must define it. It is my calling. And God is talking to me about it every day. I will tell you about a few of the pieces that I am beginning to understand, and then you can comment about other pieces that God has shown you. I want to be part of the people of God who are WHOLE and FREE!!!

I'm still working on the basics, and I will mention only two—health and finance. It is radical, and a people-think-you're-crazy act to fully surrender these two areas of life to Christ. I discovered a couple of years ago that it is a spiritual act to surrender my physical body to God and submit to His transformation. After all it is HIS house. And it is His plan to live in our bodies. He cannot accomplish His desire to transform the world if everybody is fat, sick and constantly convalescing from disease.

A month recently spent in Africa taught me that I was in bondage to food. I let it go. I am a slave of Christ, and free from all else. I will break the chains to physical need for food through fasting and redefining what food is. I will fuel my body with nourishment. I will not be enslaved and addicted to my taste buds, but it has been a process--a work of health that began, like you, with a 40 day allotment. Since then I have learned this truth:

- 70 percent of our food has been genetically modified or [GM] since 2005
- GM food damages the gut
- 80 percent of the body's immunity is in the gut

I am working to eliminate the big 4 GM foods—corn, soy, sugar beets, and canola oil. Read the labels. High fructose corn syrup, soy lecithin, and sugar are in every box of processed foods in the middle aisles of the grocery. I ask myself, "Why do half the children in the US have a chronic illness?" I don't talk about this much, because very few people are willing to surrender their food to God, but I have submitted because God wants me to be whole and free. I will pay the financial and emotional cost to stop comforting myself with false food, and fuel my body for energy. It's a resource I can give to God.

This year I have surrendered my finances more fully to God. I sold my big house on the lake, and I am positioning myself to have fewer financial pressures, and more to make available to God for His plans. How will He save a nation that has forgotten Him? How will He heal and provide and direct and show His kindness and favor? I will never know if my focus is on myself. Has anybody heard from God lately about these things? Who is talking about God's desires and God's plans? I want in on it!

God gives us richly ALL things to enjoy (I Timothy 6:17), but we only have three things to give back to Him— time, money, and energy. If you want in on this adventure, you've got to get all three in order, or you'll just be in neutral expecting the church and God to fix your needs, with no idea of God's dreams. I don't want to drift. The stakes are too high. I will make my body a living sacrifice. I will give my time and money over to the future God dreams of, not what I dream of. Will you join Him too?

Health Lesson:

Tomorrow we will begin protein meal replacements that will change your health! Today I want you to think about avoiding hunger. Here are some suggestions for success:

Add a snack between every meal!

- 10:00 a.m. - A Granny Smith apple sprinkled with stevia and cinnamon.
- 2:00 p.m. - An extra protein bar or a lettuce wrap stuffed with sugar-free salsa, 1/2 cup black beans, and 1/2 an avocado.
- 7:00 p.m. - A cup of raw or steamed carrots, cauliflower or broccoli--or a cup of all three!

Hunger is discouraging. If you work long hours, keep ziplocks of healthy low calorie snacks to keep you going. Plan an energy booster for your afternoon slump.

I want you to look in the mirror right now and be excited about what you're about to do! It's not just weight loss. You are regulating your blood pressure, decreasing cholesterol, improving kidney and liver function, eliminating toxins from your body, preventing cancer, stabilizing your blood sugar, supporting hormone balance, maximizing brain function, decreasing inflammation and helping your body use its energy more efficiently! So let's get to work.

WHAT TO DO:

Mix up a week's worth of protein bars using the following recipe —

- 2 cups chocolate protein powder
- 2 cups vanilla protein powder
- ¼ cup almond butter
- 1 15 oz can coconut milk (first pressing, no additives)

Mix in a large food processor or by hand and press into a 9 X 13 pan. Cut into 20 bars and refrigerate. Each bar is 75 calories. Two bars and a serving of fruit is a meal. Bars may be wrapped and frozen for a quick grab and go.

TIME TO WEIGH IN! Using the chart on page 154, record your initial weight and measurements (in inches) at the belly button and 2 inches below. You will not be asked to share your numbers with anyone else. I recommend weighing first thing in the morning with as few clothes on as possible. You will be recording your measurements every week to track your progress. Weigh at the same time each week and take your measurements in the same place.

Go back to your Getting Started Handout from the very first day and read it again. You'll find you have learned so much about WHY you will be eating healthy clean food that is good for your body. Have you bought everything you need for week 1? Write down your questions. Lots of people are thinking about the same thing, and you can bring them to your group when you meet this week.

Food Journal - *What I ate today:*

_____

_____

_____

_____

_____

_____

_____

Comments - *How did I feel today & what did I learn?*

_____

_____

_____

_____

_____

_____

_____

_____

What do I need to work on:

_____

_____

_____

_____

_____

_____

_____

_____

Day 12
Time to Eat

And when the tempter came to him, he said, If thou be the Son of God, command these stones to be made bread. But He answered and said, It is written, Man shall not live by bread alone, but by every word that proceedeth out of the mouth of God. Matthew 4:3-4

All things are lawful unto me, but all things are not expedient: all things are lawful for me, but I will not be brought under the power of any.
I Corinthians 6:12

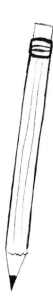

Jesus' first temptation in the wilderness was about eating, which speaks to us today about the spiritual battle that we too will fight regarding our appetite for food. Jesus had not eaten for forty days, and He needed food. He had emptied Himself of His divinity when He came to earth as a man, and He experienced all of the confines a body creates. A primary limitation of the body is that it must have fuel to function. So why didn't Jesus just do what the devil suggested? There was nothing wrong with eating bread. His need was great. His fatigue was real. Hunger was driving His mind and body at that moment. What was the moral decision involved? Just eat Jesus! You're human. Take care of your needs!

Jesus lays down a great principle in His response to appetite. He was not free to grab for food and eat just because of His hunger. EVERY aspect of His life was submitted to the Father. He would say and do only what God directed. And His first act of submission in the depths of this spiritual war was to surrender to His Father His appetite for food.

Are we called to do less? We have food all around us. It is available to us 24 hours a day in overabundance. We can have it NOW. Jesus could have had it NOW as well. But in His sinless mind and heart, He took the most basic need of His human life, and surrendered it to God. We are called to be like Him. We will not live by bread alone, but by God's words that are more essential to life than the hunger and cravings that drive our routine.

I have broken the vicious cycle of junk eating that shoots my energy levels up and crashes them an hour later. I will deny myself the pleasure of taste that is stimulated to new heights by concentrated sugars and extraordinary processed dainties that call to my pleasure centers. Let my food be ordinary. Let my food be simple. Until my soul yearns for God more than my mouth salivates for rich desserts, let me wait, as Jesus did, to hear from the Father, and to submit to Him, even my need for food. If I could relinquish the pleasure of food, perhaps He could trust me to greater kingdom work that a healthy body and a clear mind focused and laid down to His every word could accomplish.

I want to know. I want to do. Like Jesus taught through His temptation in the wilderness, and like Paul declared, all things are lawful for me, and certainly that includes the food my body needs. But it is time to see the great power food has over all of us, and bring its attraction into absolute subjection to God, whose words we will not hear until we have submitted to Him our ravenous and out-of-control desire for bread. Jesus is the model. We live in a wilderness surrounded by foods that are destroying our health. Let us be famished for God alone.

Health Lesson:

Today we will begin our Protein replacement meal program!!! Your pantry is cleaned out of "junk" – processed foods, condiments full of flavor enhancers, welcome to eating from "scratch."

Your fridge and freezer are full of clean nutrition, and your mini-blender sits on the counter ready to go. Two meals a day will be a satisfying detoxing protein shake, made with plant-based vegan protein containing a complete amino acid profile.

Compare your protein shake to the whey/soy protein supplements on your grocery store shelf by reading the attached summary. When you give your body the protein it needs, you will enjoy a curbed appetite and increased energy. Whey and soy proteins have serious drawbacks.

Let's also take a look at the other supplements you can and should add – fiber, a digestive enzyme, Omega 3s, and don't forget minerals to make you peaceful. As you learn more about nutrition you will grow in understanding of how to get what your body needs with the right amount of caloric intake. Each plays a unique role in helping you reach your maximum health potential.

WHAT TO DO:

You'll be out the door in two minutes this morning with your protein shake, full of frozen berries and a handful of spinach.

Take a Granny Smith apple, sliced and sprinkled with stevia and cinnamon, and two protein bars, or a shaker cup with protein powder for lunch.

Then for dinner, enjoy a satisfying meal of 4 ounces of healthy meat, plenty of fresh vegetables, a salad with greens, shredded vegetables, a boiled egg, black beans, avocado, etc. Choose a fat free homemade salad dressing from a recipe in the back of the book. If you don't have salad dressing already made, a little walnut oil or avocado oil with lemon and a little salt is all you need – simple and good. Keep a small supply of almonds or walnuts in your car in a closable bag. Nuts make great snacks to tide you over when you are late for a meal and hungry. You can add a protein bar for a between meal snack if needed. Keep close track of what you are eating the first few days. Stay in the window of 1,000 to 1,200 calories, adjusting upward for those who are doing physical labor at work or have a regular workout routine.

Review pages 5-8 for recipes, grocery lists and food suggestions.

7 Simple Steps
to Get Started

1. Go shopping and get prepared. Get rid of all temptations in your kitchen and replace the items with healthy choices. Let your friends and family know what you're doing so that they can support you!

2. Water is your best friend. Drink at least eight, 8 oz. glasses of water per day. If you get hungry between meals drink detox tea or broth.

3. DO NOT go more than 6 hours without having a meal. Eat every 2.5-3 hours, but remember to snack smart!

4. If you just finished working out, have a "recovery" protein shake to tide you over until your next meal.

5. Do not over eat at meals. Take your time eating to let your stomach tell you when you are actually full. No second servings.

6. Track your success. Continue to keep a food journal and record how you feel at the end of each day, using the note sections in this workbook.

7. Do not obsess over your weight. Only weigh yourself once per week, not everyday.

Q&A

What if I'm hungry?

- Make sure you get a fist size amount of protein at each meal.
- If your protein source is a shake, make sure you eat an abundance of non-starchy vegetables.
- Drink plenty of water.
- Drink your snacks - have water, detox tea or broth.

Why am I not losing weight?

- Some people do not lose weight until the 3rd week - stay with it!
- Be sure you are not loading up too many calories in the protein shakes.
- Eat plenty of non-starchy vegetables.

Why do I feel bloated after my shakes?

- Reduce the amount of fiber supplement you are using.
- Make sure you have a good probiotic as one of your supplements.

What if I'm losing weight, but I don't want to?

- Add more calories and fat to your shakes.
- Eat any fruit.
- Add a starchy carb to your meals such as brown rice.
- Put an extra scoop of protein in your shakes.

What if I'm constipated?

- Make sure you are drinking at least 64oz. of water per day.
- Vegetables, vegetables, vegetables!
- Add ground flax seed or selium

Whey/Soy Protein vs. Pea Vegetable Protein
Is Your Protein Helping or Hurting You?

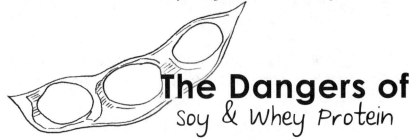

The Dangers of
Soy & Whey Protein

SOY

- Highly allergenic (regardless of the method of process)

- Low incorporation levels

- Contains phytoestrogens (can lead to estrogen dominance)

- Can cause fatigue, weight gain, insomnia, increase risk for chronic disease, feminization in men

WHEY

- Highly allergenic (not just "milk" allergy)

- Hard to digest

- Can deposit in intestinal tract and colon

- Can lead to long term kidney and liver damage

Choose a vegan protein that includes a complete amino acid profile, high in Glutamine, Arginine, Lysine, Luecine, and branch chain amino acids. How it is extracted is as important as its nutrient content. Using a cold extrusion process, the protein must be free of solvents, GMOs, radiation, artificial colors, and preservatives, flavors, herbicides, and pesticides.

Using a vegan protein naturally avoids the most common allergens, dairy, egg, gluten, soy, added sugar, wheat, or yeast.

Protein will assist you in building muscle, managing weight, curbing appetite, raising metabolism and blowing the roof off your energy level all while improving your overall health.

Raw Pea Protein

Peas are a high fiber, low calorie, nutrient dense vegetable-based SUPERFOOD, and also a remarkable source of plant-based proteins and amino acids! The amino acids found in peas include Lysine, Arginine, Glutamine, Leucine, Isoleucine & Valine (Branched Chain Amino Acids - BCAAs)and:

- Aid muscle tissue maintenance
- Compares to egg and milk proteins
- BCAAs are higher in pea protein than any other vegetable protein
- Helps restore nitrogen balance after intense physiological stress
- Increases muscle mass while reducing body fat during intense exercise
- Improves vasodilation and promotes a healthy heart
- Assists in maintaining lean body mass

- Facilitates calcium absorption (promoting healthy bone development in children)
- Boosts the immune system: producing antibodies, hormones, enzymes, collagen, and tissue-repair
- Low in sulfur proteins (sulfur proteins speed up the aging process)
- Increases metabolism and satiety (helping you to feel "full")
- Natural tonic for preventing and treating high blood pressure
- Promotes healthy kidney function

The proteins naturally present in peas exist in an inactive state and must be activated by special enzymes to become bio-available. Simply consuming peas will not provide the same health benefits as using a purified pea protein extract.

Raw Cranberry Protein

To the pea protein find a protein that adds cranberry protein. It is unique in that it is the only 100% plant protein that contains 25% complete protein including all essential amino acids.

The extraction of the cranberry protein should use cold-pressing technology preserving natural balances and naturally occurring fatty acids, which increases the absorption of the other nutrients. Cranberry protein is also:

- Powerful detoxifier and diuretic (flushes out the kidneys)
- Treats bladder, kidney and urinary problems
- Boosts immune system, protecting against influenza and the common cold
- Increases "good" cholesterol (HDL), and reduces "bad" cholesterol (LDL)
- Improves circulation and reduces risk of heart disease
- Helps to relieve stress & depression
- Treats skin conditions such as: acne, dermatitis, psoriasis, burns & wounds
- Also considered one of the best remedies for REDUCING CELLULITE!

Raw Rice Protein

Look for raw rice added to the pea and cranberry proteins to complete the amino acid profile adding the 9 amino acids your body cannot produce on its own. Rice protein is whole grain. Whole grain and foods made from them contain all the essential parts and natural-occurring nutrients of the entire grain seed.

The rice protein contained in your vegan protein should be organic. So look for a protein from natural, clean sources. It is excellent for your heart health according the food and drug administration. It is allergen free, soy free and gluten free and that's especially good for people either on a gluten free diet or someone with Celiac Disease.

Look for a protein with no ingredients cooked or heated. When ingredients are cooked or heated the nutrient content is damaged or lost. What you see is what you get. All raw ingredients, that contain their true nutritional content, are perfect for vegans on a raw diet.

Why Is Protein So Important For My Regular Diet?

Protein is essential for growth and repair and makes up about 15% of the mass of the average person. Much of the human body is constructed from protein molecules, which play a crucial role in virtually all of the body's biological processes. Amino acids are the building blocks of protein and the body produces them naturally, except for nine essential amino acids. This means the body does not make them and must consume these amino acids from animal or plant-food sources.

How Much Protein Is Enough?

On average, a healthy adult needs 1 gram of protein per 2.2lbs of body weight per day (roughly half your body weight). For example, an adult weighing 150 pounds would need 70 grams per day divided between meals for basic nutrition.

The health regimen in this workbook is designed primarily for weight loss via protein shakes for 2 out of 3 meals each day for 30 days. You will need enough protein to make two shakes per day, each containing around 20 grams of protein. Add a good source of soluble fiber to increase your daily fiber intake and assist your liver in detoxing as your body reduces.

Healthy Weight and Muscle Gain

For active men and women who regularly exercise, protein consumed within an hour after working out will provide amino acids for the building and repair of muscle tissue. If you wish to gain weight (especially muscle mass), simply continue eating normal meals and add the protein supplements ideally after the workout session for muscle recovery.

Weight Management

If weight maintenance is your goal, protein shakes make a great breakfast or lunch on the go; add fruits or veggies to make a smoothie.

Healthy Shakes For Children

Children also benefit from protein shakes, particularly when included in smoothies made with whole foods like spinach, kale, berries, avocado, or banana. For a child weighing 30 pounds, the recommended serving would be approximately 5 grams of protein powder added to a smoothie with added spinach, avocado, berries, etc.

Got Protein?

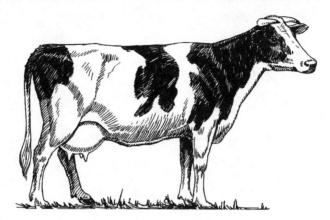

Whey Facts:

- Whey is a by-product of the cheese making process
- Dairy cows are loaded with hormones and antibiotics
- Whey is highly processed
- High in cholesterol
- Highly acidic causing inflammation in the body
- Highly allergenic and difficult to digest
- Most brands contain artificial flavors, colors and sweeteners
- Consumer Reports June 1, 2010 investigation found contaminants and heavy metals in the top whey protein powders and ready made drinks

What to Look for in a Quality Protein Supplement:

- Vegan protein from brown rice, yellow peas or cranberries
- Added vitamins and minerals for a complete meal replacement
- Dairy, gluten and soy free
- No artificial flavors, colors or sweeteners
- Non-allergenic
- Easily digestible and absorbable
- No cholesterol, no GMO and a low glycemic index

Food Journal - *What I ate today:*

_____

_____

_____

_____

_____

_____

_____

Comments - *How did I feel today & what did I learn?*

_____

_____

_____

_____

_____

_____

_____

_____

What do I need to work on:

_____

_____

_____

_____

_____

_____

_____

_____

Day 13

God's Saving Health for the Nations

God be merciful unto us, and bless us, and cause His face to shine upon us; that thy way may be known upon the earth, and thy saving health among all nations... God shall bless us; and all the ends of the earth shall fear Him." Psalm 67:1-2, 7

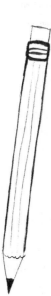

God has a great purpose in giving His children knowledge, understanding, and health. How lavish will God be in blessing me? It has to be pretty extravagant to get the attention of the ends of the earth! The world should see Christians as the extraordinarily blessed, so supernaturally healthy, and full of provision, and joyfully surrounded by family and friends, that they would be drawn to our God! How can they know if we do not have better health than the pagans, or greater love for one another, or blessing and favor from God?

God's great gifts are everywhere around me, and as His child I want to honor my Father by caring for the gifts He has given. He smiles when I polish the red oak floors I asked Him for. He is pleased when I run on my treadmill and eat carefully to protect the health He has lavished on me. Why would I ever waste those things or dishonor Him by treating them as having no value? They are the symbols of blessing and favor and honor that my Father is pleased to give to me.

He asks me to seek His kingdom while He adds more to my life. Look at me world! I walk in the supernatural favor of Almighty God! My life is a demonstration of God's perfect faithfulness, protection, and provision. And you can experience His great moment-by-moment kindness and generosity too. Will you do your part to nurture your body as a witness to all nations of God's saving health?

Health Lesson:

Hormone Balance will help you lose weight and return your body to optimal health. *Dr. Deanna's Healing Handbook* explains the benefit of bioidentical progesterone in the treatment of hormone imbalance for both men and women. Chapter 2 of her book is an in depth explanation of the how and why of hormone balance. This is critical for weight loss and health management.

For Women:

Hormones get out of balance through a variety of factors including dietary consumption of false estrogens, lifestyle, medications, and even environment. Diet plays a big role. A diet high in carbohydrates or simple sugars will make hormonal imbalance worse.

When you are consuming a diet high in carbohydrates your body's response is to have high circulating insulin levels. High insulin levels can be deleterious because insulin is a growth hormone and it is the only hormone in the body that causes us to store fat in fat cells. Estrogen can also be produced in fat cells, even if a woman has had a hysterectomy and can give men female features. A high carbohydrate diet packs on weight around the waist in particular further contributing to hormone imbalance. See Dr. Deanna's recommendation for the application of 20mg of topical bioidentical progesterone cream daily for women not menstruating, for those menstruating, 20mg after ovulation for 10-12 days until menstruation. Some conditions require adjustments, see Chapter 2 of *Dr. Deanna's Healing Handbook* for further guidance.

For Men:

It is well known that the estradiol level in 55-year old men, for example, is usually a bit higher than that of a 55-year old woman. Prostate cancer occurs, in part, because testosterone and progesterone levels fall with age and estrogen levels rise, leading to estrogen dominance in older men.

Of the three estrogens, estradiol in particular is harmful to a man's prostate because it causes the prostate to enlarge and likely is one of the main causes of prostate cancer. Like women, men are often prescribed diuretics and other pharmaceuticals to address prostate enlargement and the resulting frequent urination, without getting to the root of the hormone imbalance.

Progesterone is a precursor and regulator for the production of testosterone. Progesterone inhibits the conversion of testosterone to di-hydro-testosterone (DHT) just like the drug, Proscar® and Saw Palmetto, except progesterone is a much more potent inhibitor of this detrimental conversion. It is recommended to use 5-10 mg. of bioidentical topical progesterone cream daily.

WHAT TO DO:

Eat clean foods free of pesticides and chemical preservatives (false estrogens), which can interfere with hormone imbalance. Consider a bioidentical progesterone supplement if you have symptoms of hormone balance.

Make sure the products you are putting on your skin are not false estrogens (mineral oil, parabens, phthalates) getting absorbed into the bloodstream.

Eat balanced snacks or meals that include whole foods containing protein, complex carbohydrates, healthy and high quality fats, and fiber.

Have a protein shake with added fiber for breakfast, two protein bars and a Granny Smith apple sprinkled with stevia for lunch, and a healthy dinner of 4 oz. lean meat, plenty of vegetables, and a salad with homemade good oil (walnut, coconut, or avocado oil) dressing.

If you are struggling with hunger, save a hundred calories for a between meal snack. See A Sample Day on page 34 for suggestions.

Food Journal - *What I ate today:*

_____

_____

_____

_____

_____

_____

_____

Comments - *How did I feel today & what did I learn?*

_____

_____

_____

_____

_____

_____

_____

_____

What do I need to work on:

_____

_____

_____

_____

_____

_____

_____

Day 14

Jesus Understands the Need for Food

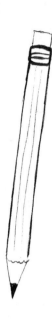

Then Jesus called his disciples unto him, and said, I have compassion on the multitude, because they continue with me now three days, and have nothing to eat: and I will not send them away fasting, lest they faint in the way. Matthew 15:32

The hunger of 4,000 people in the wilderness gives us opportunity to understand the depth of Jesus' concern and sympathy for us. He cared about the nourishment of their bodies. Their appetite for the things of God had placed them in difficulty. For three days they had attended closely to his teaching, and chose to set aside their own agenda to value Jesus' agenda. There was no food in the wilderness for such a multitude. When we nurture our appetite for God by seeking him above all other things that vie for our attention, we too are placed in a position of blessing. Jesus tenderly responds to their need for food, not willing that they should be famished, either in body or in soul. Neither does He leave us weary and unfed to find our way alone. We will realign the priority of our appetites in this transition to health, and we will find, as the 4,000 did, that the Holy Spirit of compassion will not send us away, but will nourish our souls and our bodies because our hearts long to submit our appetites to His Lordship. Expect a miracle! Your body will be changed, and your heart will be changed. Jesus will minister to all of our needs.

Health Lesson:

I read an article recently about the state of American health care, and how it will not give us the health and long life we need. We spent twice as much as any nation in the world on health care, and are ranked last in quality of health of developed nations. Here is a list of six things we can do to take control of our health. I am committed to getting healthy, and helping as many people as I can avoid the "big four" diet related diseases--cancer, heart disease, high blood pressure, and diabetes. This 40 day prgoram has changed my life. I hope you are enjoying the diet and how you are beginning to feel.

Dr. Mercola gives us a summary of the major components of a healthy lifestyle in the following excerpt:

Most of the Leading Causes of Death are Preventable

The majority of deaths are due to chronic, not acute, disease. And most chronic diseases, including cancer, heart disease, diabetes, and obesity, are largely preventable with simple lifestyle changes.

Even infectious diseases like the flu can often be warded off by a healthy way of life. Just imagine the lowered death toll, not to mention costs to the economy, if more people decided to take control of their health … heart disease and cancer alone accounted for 47 percent of deaths in the United States in 2010, and there are many strategies you can implement to lower your risk of these diseases.

Proper Food Choices

Generally speaking, you should be looking to focus your diet on whole, ideally organic, unprocessed foods that come from healthy, sustainable, ideally local, sources. Sugar, and fructose in particular, can act as a toxin in and of itself when consumed in excess, and as such drive multiple disease processes in your body, not the least of which is insulin resistance, a major cause of accelerated aging and virtually all chronic disease.

Comprehensive Exercise Program, including High-Intensity Exercise

Even if you're eating the healthiest diet in the world, you still need to exercise to reach the highest levels of health, and you need to be exercising effectively, which means including not only core-strengthening exercises, strength training, and stretching but also high-intensity activities into your rotation.

Stress Reduction

You cannot be optimally healthy if you avoid addressing the emotional component of your health and longevity, as your emotional state plays a role in nearly every physical disease -- from heart disease and depression, to arthritis and cancer. Prayer, gratitude, and scheduled leisure time should be a part of your daily life.

Optimize Vitamin D with Proper Sun Exposure

We have long known that it is best to get your vitamin D from appropriate sun exposure during times when UVB rays are present. Vitamin D plays an important role in preventing numerous illnesses ranging from cancer to the flu.

Be aware that if you take supplemental vitamin D, you also need to make sure you're getting enough vitamin K2, as these two nutrients work in tandem to ensure calcium is distributed into the proper areas in your body. Vitamin K2 deficiency is actually what produces the symptoms of vitamin D toxicity, which includes inappropriate calcification that can lead to hardening of your arteries.

High Quality Animal-Based Omega-3 Fats

Animal-based omega-3 fat like krill oil is a strong factor in helping people live longer, and many experts believe that it is likely the predominant reason why the Japanese are the longest lived race on the planet.

Avoid as Many Chemicals, Toxins, and Pollutants as Possible

This includes tossing out your toxic household cleaners, soaps, personal hygiene products, air fresheners, bug sprays, lawn pesticides, and insecticides, just to name a few, and replacing them with non-toxic alternatives.

WHAT TO DO:

It is always good to review the steps you have taken towards health. The following are three lists you have seen before. Read through them carefully, and circle any suggestions you have yet to practice in your daily routine:

- Cleansing List (Day 5)
- Sample Day (Day 9)
- 7 Steps to Get Started (Day 12)

These lists seemed overwhelming the first time you saw them. Now as you choose to take more steps toward health, don't forget to say, "Thank you, God. Look how far we have come!"

Cleansing List

ELIMINATE:

- Alcohol
- Artificial sweeteners
- Beef that is not grassfed
- Coffee
- Corn
- Dairy
- Non cage-free eggs
- Farm-raised fish
- All fruit EXCEPT limes, lemons, green apples & berries
- Gluten
- Nitrates
- MSG
- Peanuts & peanut butter
- Pork
- Soy
- Sugar, honey & maple syrup
- Vinegar
- White potatoes

INCLUDE:

- Almond, coconut & flax milk
- Almond butter
- Almonds (raw), walnuts & pecans
- Avocado
- Beef, grassfed (1x per week)
- Brown rice
- Chicken and turkey, free-range
- Coconut sugar
- Eggs, cage-free
- Green & herb teas
- Legumes
- Non starchy vegetables
- Organic green apples & berries
- Olive, avocado, coconut & walnut oil
- Quinoa
- Stevia or Xylitol
- Sweet potatoes, yams & turnips
- Wild-caught, cold water fish (1x per week)

A Sample Day
with An Appetite for God

Wake Up
Cup of Detox Tea or Organic Coffee (if you need caffeine first thing)

Breakfast
Protein Shake with fiber supplement and probiotics.

Snack (optional)
Granny Smith apple sprinkled with stevia and cinnamon, protein bar, raw vegetables, small handful of nuts, seeds, or a tsp. of almond butter.

Lunch (4 hours after breakfast)
2 protein bars and a Granny Smith apple
- or -
A green salad topped with boiled eggs, black beans, vegetables and home made dressing.

Snack (optional)
See above

Dinner
A fist size of a lean protein, non-starchy veggies, a green salad topped with boiled eggs, black beans, vegetables and home made dressing. and a small amount of healthy fat.

DO NOT EAT AFTER 7PM!
Have a cup of detox tea if you get hungry.

Recovery Shake
If you work out intensely for an hour or more, make sure you have a recovery shake within 30 minutes of completing your workout. Your next meal will be within 4 hours when you become hungry. The recovery shake is in addition to your healthy meal plan.

Circle the steps and suggestions below you need to work on.

7 Simple Steps
to Get started

1. Go shopping and get prepared. Get rid of all temptations in your kitchen and replace the items with healthy choices. Let your friends and family know what you're doing so that they can support you!

2. Water is your best friend. Drink at least eight, 8 oz. glasses of water per day. If you get hungry between meals drink detox tea or broth.

3. DO NOT go more than 6 hours without having a meal. Eat every 2.5-3 hours, but remember to snack smart!

4. If you just finished working out, have a "recovery" protein shake to tide you over until your next meal.

5. Do not over eat at meals. Take your time eating to let your stomach tell you when you are actually full. No second servings.

6. Track your success. Continue to keep a food journal and record how you feel at the end of each day, using the note sections in this workbook.

7. Do not obsess over your weight. Only weigh yourself once per week, not everyday.

Q&A

What if I'm hungry?

- Make sure you get a fist size amount of protein at each meal.
- If your protein source is a shake, make sure you eat an abundance of non-starchy vegetables.
- Drink plenty of water.
- Drink your snacks - have water, detox tea or broth.

Why am I not losing weight?

- Some people do not lose weight until the 3rd week - stay with it!
- Be sure you are not loading up too many calories in the protein shakes.
- Eat plenty of non-starchy vegetables.

Why do I feel bloated after my shakes?

- Reduce the amount of fiber supplement you are using.
- Make sure you have a good probiotic as one of your supplements.

What if I'm losing weight, but I don't want to?

- Add more calories and fat to your shakes.
- Eat any fruit.
- Add a starchy carb to your meals such as brown rice.
- Put an extra scoop of protein in your shakes.

What if I'm constipated?

- Make sure you are drinking at least 64oz. of water per day.
- Vegetables, vegetables, vegetables!
- Add ground flax seed or selium

Food Journal - *What I ate today:*

_____

_____

_____

_____

_____

_____

_____

_____

Comments - *How did I feel today & what did I learn?*

_____

_____

_____

_____

_____

_____

_____

_____

_____

What do I need to work on:

_____

_____

_____

_____

_____

_____

_____

_____

_____

Day 15

Healthy in Soul and Body

Beloved, I wish above all things that thou mayest prosper and be in health, even as thy soul prospereth. For I rejoiced greatly, when the brethren came and testified of the truth that is in thee, even as thou walkest in the truth. I have no greater joy than to hear that my children walk in truth. 3 John 1:2-4

John's message here is a most direct reference to the importance of physical health. He wanted his friend's physical health to equal his spiritual fervor. We are often criticized for putting the importance of physical health on a high spiritual plane, but John, in his later years, wisely understood and addresses the issue.

Physical health is a great gift of God, and we need to tend His treasure carefully. John also acknowledges here the connection between the physical body, the soul and the mind. A sick, toxic, sluggish, overweight body has a direct influence on the mind and soul. Your sense of well being, your understanding of what is real and true, even your spiritual perceptions of how God is at work are greatly influenced by the state of your body.

May we take our physical fitness seriously, not mistakenly thinking the only thing that matters is our soul fitness! We have Kingdom work to do! May your body and soul prosper together, and may your mind grasp the truth about your health!

Health Lesson:

So why detoxify...how does it help you?

Our body is like a bathtub, the water faucet (brings toxins in), and the drain (lets the toxins out). When it is running at a normal pace, we don't have much of a problem. When we are in overload and the drain is plugged, the tub gradually fills up and spills over the sides. This is when people get sick and you are given a mop (medicine) which can also add even more toxins and have side effects.

We believe most people want to lose weight and feel good but they don't really understand how to achieve true health and vitality. Toxins are locked up in fat cells!

To have effective weight loss, we have to unplug the drain (detox) by nutritional cleansing. When you get rid of the toxins, the fat can melt away! Simply put, toxins come from the environment, processed foods, extra weight and being inactive. Stress leads to toxic build up which leads to inflammation. Though we are often unaware of low grade inflammation, the body's slow burn at the cellular level over time contributes to chronic disease.

Decreasing stressors/toxins will decrease inflammation, which will decrease the disease breeding ground... creating health! We want to eliminate these toxins by using detox tea and a total body cleanse. It's time to CLEAN the DRAIN!!

We recommend a Detox Tea containing milk thistle, whose unique ability to protect the liver is undisputed. Milk thistle's active ingredient helps repair damaged liver cells by stimulating protein synthesis and encouraging liver cell growth. Its potent antioxidants reduce inflammation, and has been recommended for liver disease, hepatitis, mushroom poisoning, and to detoxify and cleanse synthetic chemicals from our bodies, including heavy metals. It has also been used to treat irritable bowel syndrome, adrenal disorders and psoriasis. Milk Thistle is also found in immunity boosters, along with combination probiotics, which makes perfect sense when its function is understood. I took special notice of milk thistle because of a conversation I had with a relative last month. He has survived two serious car accidents, and takes pain medication and vitamin supplements. He told me, "milk thistle is the most important supplement I take, because it boosts the function of my liver to get rid of any supplements my body doesn't use, and protects it from damage from acetaminophen based pain medicine." Your liver is your most important cleansing organ. Give it a boost today with a delicious cup of Detox Tea!

WHAT TO DO:

Planning ahead is so essential. Always have a few protein bars in a ziplock bag and take them with you. When you are running late, it will keep you away from the fast food junk that is everywhere!

The program should be feeling routine by now. A shake for breakfast, protein bars and a piece of low glycemic fruit ("Google" your fruit to determine the glycemic index – a Granny Smith apple has a low GI like blueberries and strawberries – good antioxidants to counter inflammation in your body) for lunch, and dinner is a big salad topped with a boiled egg or black beans, carrots, tomatoes, spinach, snap peas, cucumbers, etc. Add 4 oz. of lean meat and a generous serving of steamed broccoli, cauliflower, green beans, or asparagus. Sprinkle with garlic powder. Watch out for the seasoning mixes. They contain sugar, MSG, wheat, and preservatives. Don't you love the simplicity of this program? Eat clean, eat simply – it's delicious!

NUTRITIONAL REBALANCING **IS NOT A DIET**

Fat is crearted to protect body from toxins & impurities creating unwanted weight.

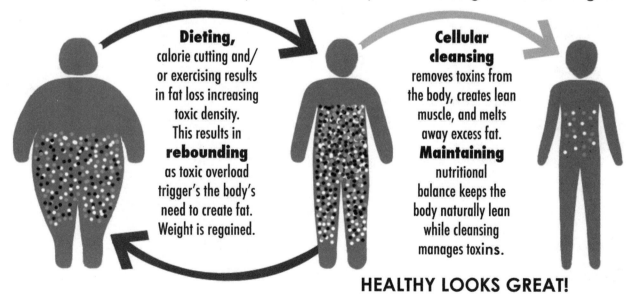

Dieting, calorie cutting and/ or exercising results in fat loss increasing toxic density. This results in **rebounding** as toxic overload trigger's the body's need to create fat. Weight is regained.

Cellular cleansing removes toxins from the body, creates lean muscle, and melts away excess fat. **Maintaining** nutritional balance keeps the body naturally lean while cleansing manages toxins.

HEALTHY LOOKS GREAT!

Food Journal - *What I ate today:*

_____

_____

_____

_____

_____

_____

_____

Comments - *How did I feel today & what did I learn?*

_____

_____

_____

_____

_____

_____

_____

_____

_____

What do I need to work on:

_____

_____

_____

_____

_____

_____

_____

_____

Day 16

Entertaining God's Way

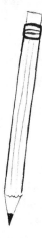

Be not forgetful to entertain strangers: for thereby some have entertained angels unawares. Hebrews 13:2

One of the hard things for me in letting go of the SAD diet was the thought of being unable to entertain. We have always enjoyed inviting people to dinner at our home, and holiday parties frequently included tables full of homemade pies, rich desserts and sugary fruit punch. Consider having a potluck at your next group meeting. Each person can bring a dish that is sugar and GMO free, grain free, and nourishing! Our home is still an open place for entertaining and we have even hosted cooking classes to help others learn how to leave the SAD diet behind for good! Instead of going to a junk food restaurant, why not invite someone over for lunch, and prepare a simple nourishing meal with meat, fruits, vegetables, nuts and seeds. You will both be amazed at how good it is to give and get the gift of health, and who knows? The Hebrew writer says you may be entertaining an angel or two along the way!

Health Lesson:

Today we are going to look at what it means to have healthy gut bacteria. Here is an excerpt from *Dr. Deanna's Healing Handbook:*

How to Improve Your Gut Health
Enzyme and Probiotic Supplements

A youthful healthy gut produces digestive enzymes such as pepsin, protease, amylase, and lipase, to break down food into the amino acids necessary for healthy metabolism. As a person ages, these enzymes decrease resulting in less than optimal digestion of foods. Probiotic bacteria are the digestion "factory" in the gut.

The common probiotics such as *Lactobacillus* are only effective for the initial breakdown of large food molecules in the stomach, since they do not survive beyond the strong acidic environment of the stomach. Unlike *Lactobacillus*, the majority of *Bifidobacteria* survive stomach acid, populating and regulating digestive activity and gut lining health in the small intestine.

A good prebiotic is a fiber that is fermented in the large intestine, and provides nourishment to feed and proliferate the probiotic bacteria. Examples are inulin and oligofructose. These stimulate the production of good bacteria in the colon to aid in stabilizing blood sugar, cholesterol, and triglycerides. Most probiotic supplements contain live cultures of different species of *Lactobacillus* and *Bifidobacteria*. See the chapter on gut health in *Dr. Deanna's Healing Handboo*k for a full explanation of probiotic benefits.

Most of us have allowed wheat gluten to create an intestinal "road rash" in our gut damaging the intestinal microvilli, interfering with absorption of key nutrients as well as detoxification of the body. In the case of the gut, if you give the body what it needs, it can often repair itself. Give your gut a good prebiotic, probiotic and digestive enzyme.

Maintain Healthy Blood Glucose Levels

Americans could accurately be described as wheat-a-holics, with a per capita consumption of 133 pounds of wheat annually. This equals a half loaf of bread per day. Today's wheat pushes blood sugar higher than other foods, it's no longer the "daily bread" for which the Lord taught us to pray. Hybridization and other well-intentioned meddling have made wheat consumption actually a health threat.

When the cycle of glucose-insulin reaches abnormal highs and lows several times a day, it provokes growth of belly fat, which is associated with insulin resistance, which leads to even higher levels of glucose and insulin, damaging pancreatic beta cells, and making the wheat addict more susceptible to diabetes (See Dr. William Davis's book, *Wheat Belly*, pp. 103-104).

Omega 3 Essential Fatty Acid Supplement

Omega 3's are a supplement that everyone should be taking for many of the body's system operations. In the gut, Omegas help with the absorption of carbs, they are used to repair gaps that occur between cells from damage caused by gluten, and they help stabilize blood sugar levels which in turn keep insulin levels low. In addition, they decrease the amount of beta amyloid protein build up in the brain. Beta amyloid is the protein that causes "tangles" in the brain and leads to Alzheimer's disease. Studies show that Omega 3's reduce the amount of beta amyloid protein. 1000 mg can reduce the beta amyloid by 30%, 2000 mg can reduce by 60%.

What about yogurt? Manufacturers of processed yogurt expose the finished product to high heat in order to shut down fermentation, which kills the bacteria, but gives the yogurt a longer shelf life. In addition, the flavored yogurts have 100% more sugar than a sugar sweetened bowl of cereal! The dry probiotic enzymes will survive the stomach's acid, because they are designed to bypass it, and become active in the intestine. Yogurt may help with constipation and give a sense of benefit because it contains a potent laxative, inulin. It is a filler and stabilizer used in processed foods, and keeps dairy products from separating. However, this yogurt product is doing nothing to enhance the gut microflora which affects every health system.

WHAT TO DO:

Avoid the GMO quartet—read every label, and do not buy any product that contains corn, soy, sugar, or canola/cottonseed oil. Buying organic foods is the right solution. You not only avoid genetically modified food, you are also avoiding pesticide sprays, antibiotics in meat, and unnecessary chemical additives that create a toxic store in your body depriving you of optimal health.

Watch a short video entitled "Gut Health" in the multimedia section of the www.AppetiteforGod.com.

Food Journal - *What I ate today:*

_____
_____
_____
_____
_____
_____
_____
_____

Comments - *How did I feel today & what did I learn?*

_____
_____
_____
_____
_____
_____
_____
_____
_____

What do I need to work on:

_____
_____
_____
_____
_____
_____
_____
_____
_____

Day 17

More Necessary Than Food

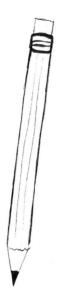

Neither have I gone back from the commandment of his lips; I have esteemed the words of his mouth more than my necessary food.
Job 23:12

Job is our great example in holding on to our faith in the midst of high-pressure adversity. How do you respond to grief and loss? Too often, food instead of reliance upon the Holy Spirit becomes the comfort we turn to when the pressures of life are pressing in, and our bad choices of sugar and processed foods add to depression, weight gain, and hormone imbalance.

If you are in a hard place in your life, ask yourself if food has become comfort rather than fuel for good health, which is so important in a time of great physical stress. You will be successful during this 40 days by "esteeming the words of His mouth." Job compares esteeming God's word--to hold in high honor the promises and commandments God has given you, to persevere, enduring the hardship of a soldier and the discipline of a son—over against the desire for necessary food.

As a nation, we need to examine our necessary food. Psalm 105:16 describes a famine in Israel: *Moreover he called for a famine upon the land: he brake the whole staff of bread.* A 16th century commentator writes that the famine occurred, "either by sending scarcity, or by taking away the strength and nourishment thereof." Our current hybridized wheat has without question had its strength and nourishment removed so that the whole staff of our bread is broken. We have modified and processed the grain until we live in a famine evidenced by a plague of chronic disease and obesity. A warning from Leviticus sounds like the modern bakery had its roots in very ancient times--

> *And when I have broken the staff of your bread, ten women shall bake your bread in one oven, and they shall deliver you your bread again by weight: and ye shall eat, and not be satisfied.*

Let us be content and satisfied with "our necessary food," fuel for making our bodies fit and healthy, and let the focus of our hearts be upon "the words of His mouth."

Health Lesson:

Anyone who eats nonorganic meat is exposed to antibiotics. Unless specifically labeled otherwise, beef, chicken, turkey and farm raised fish are regularly fed antibiotics as well as genetically modified corn. In fact, eighty percent of all antibiotics in the U.S. are consumed by food animals. Antibiotics cause permanent damage to the gut flora and leave our immune systems compromised. They are especially troublesome for young children who need a strong gut immunity to overcome the toxic effects of 49 scheduled doses of vaccines before age six.

Although all antibiotics compromise gut immunity, the quinolones Cipro and Levaquin have the most reported side effects. They are neurotoxic, causing frequent peripheral and central nervous system difficulties. Joint pain, especially in the hips, elbows, wrists, and ankles is common. The pain is often severe, and can last for months or years. If you or a loved one are prescribed these drugs, research the effects of fluoroquinolone toxicity on the internet before taking them. These drugs are not recommended for anyone who has symptoms of an autoimmune disorder such as Celiac, Crohns, lupus, or multiple sclerosis.

Originally intended for the treatment of Anthrax, fluoroquinolones are now used for minor infections such as urinary tract and sinus infections. If you struggle with urinary tract infections, research the benefits of the simple sugar D-Mannose. The body metabolizes a small percentage of it, and *E. coli* are attracted to the sugar and excreted. *E. coli* cause 90 percent of UTI's. Taking a D-Mannose sugar pill each day can prevent *E. coli* overgrowth. Colloidal silver solution is also recommended by naturopaths as an alternative to antibiotics. Food and environmental allergies can be eliminated aiding in the avoidance of sinus and ear infections and the need for antibiotics.

Disclaimer: These suggestions are for educational purposes only and are not meant as medical advice.

WHAT TO DO:

Watch a short video entitled "Antibiotics in Meat", then write down your questions to discuss with your group. To watch the video go to multimedia section of the www.AppetiteforGod.com.

Browse a website or Pinterest board of Paleo main dishes and choose one to add to your meal plan.

If you haven't bought your 7-day cleanse yet, buy one to be ready to start on Day 19. Use a high quality whole body detoxifier that cleanses the blood and major organs as well as the colon.

When you go shopping check tomato products and beans—no sugar, no MSG! It's amazing what they add sugar to. Read every label. Costco sells organic tomatoes, sauce, and paste for less than non-organics at the grocery. Organic is always the right choice!

Food Journal - *What I ate today:*

_____

_____

_____

_____

_____

_____

_____

Comments - *How did I feel today & what did I learn?*

_____

_____

_____

_____

_____

_____

_____

_____

_____

What do I need to work on:

_____

_____

_____

_____

_____

_____

_____

Day 18

Is Exercise Important?

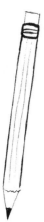

Exercise thyself rather unto Godliness. I Timothy 4:7

The 4th chapter of First Timothy is often misquoted to prove that people shouldn't worry about food or exercise. Paul understood the bondage of a set of rules that demanded things like abstaining from meat or exercising. So he told Timothy to have an appetite for God. He was to make his desires align with the "nourishment of faith and good doctrine." However, many people cannot nourish their faith because they have failed to fuel their bodies for health. We become derailed from God's plan when we have no strength. Daniel said of God's people, ***"but the people that do know their God shall be strong, and do exploits"*** (Daniel 11:32). We will fuel our bodies to have the strength and energy to pursue the spiritual exercise that brings Godliness. It takes work to avoid nutrition-depleted cheap food that appeals so powerfully to our taste. Food appetites that are harmful to our bodies are also harmful to our calling to be strong, do exploits for God, and find freedom in the Spirit.

Health Lesson:

Weight control is 85 percent diet and 15 percent exercise. A moderate exercise program during the Appetite for God program is encouraged. Walk a mile. Moderate aerobics and stretching are great! However, your body will be going through some drastic changes over the next several days and all excess energy will be wrapped up in the detoxifying process (your gut primarily). Therefore, we recommend light exercise during the first days of your detox. Heavy exercise will leave you completely exhausted and might also sabotage your weight loss goals. At all times, you want to make sure your net caloric intake (food calories minus exercise calories) is around 1000 to 1200. If you fall below this mark, your body will go into 'store' or 'starve' mode and will hold on to weight, instead of lose it.

Listen to your body. Be mindful of expenditure and compensate with approved snacks or adding more calories to your shakes. Also, if your exercise session is high intensity and over 60 minutes in duration, you are allowed (and highly encouraged) to have a "recovery shake". This shake CAN include higher sugar fruits i.e. banana, pineapple, mango, etc. At some point, you might find yourself thinking... "I will run for a banana these days!"

WHAT TO DO:

TIME TO WEIGH IN! Using the chart on page 154, continue to record your weight and measurements. Weigh at the same time each week and measure in the same places every time. Exercise and fitness is a great boon to the immune system, mood, blood circulation and outwardly beautiful skin. Walk one mile with a friend today. Begin every morning with ten minutes of stretching exercises.

It's time to go grocery shopping! Make a list – be prepared. Have you noticed how much less you spend on groceries when you eat simpler? I thought it would be so expensive to eat healthy, but my grocery bill dropped dramatically when I started this healthy eating program. Spend an hour browsing Kroger's organic section or visit a health food store. Read the labels, not everything in health food stores is good for you. Buy plenty of fresh or frozen organic vegetables. They are very low in calories, and you can use them as snacks. Avoid anything in a box or a can. You can save money by buying bulk organic frozen fruits and vegetables at a member store like Costco or Sam's Club. When your group gets together, have someone compile a list of shopping tips that apply to your local stores, farmer's markets, and cooperatives.

Food Journal - *What I ate today:*

_____

_____

_____

_____

_____

_____

Comments - *How did I feel today & what did I learn?*

_____

_____

_____

_____

_____

_____

_____

What do I need to work on:

_____

_____

_____

_____

_____

_____

_____

Day 19

The Cost of Dainty Desserts

Two things have I required of thee; deny me them not before I die: Remove far from me vanity and lies: give me neither poverty nor riches; feed me with food convenient for me: Lest I be full, and deny thee, and say, Who is the Lord? or lest I be poor, and steal, and take the name of my God in vain. Proverbs 30:7-9

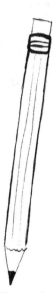

Many in America can't imagine what it is like to be so hungry we would steal for food, but most of us have sat down to a dinner and eaten until we were more than FULL!

Thanksgiving dinner in our family for half a century was all about the homemade pies. They weren't convenient food—it took a full day to make them in preparation for the ritual that would stuff us fatter than the turkey. Our appetite for food gets out of control so easily.

Solomon knew the danger of making rich, complicated, unnatural foods the center of life. I have been there. I have forgotten that God is the one who feeds me. He has chosen my days, my place of birth, and my family and He has designed my body to be nourished with food planted in His garden full of essential amino and fatty acids.

I am thankful for the tradition of prayer before each and every meal. We need to be reminded of the Giver, and let go of our appetites that fill us up with addictive sugar, but leave us craving more. I want convenient food. Like filling up my car at the gas station. Our cars have an "energy" tank for gas and we would never over fill it. Adequate fuel makes it useful for work and productivity just as our eating to fill our "energy" tanks should.

Fill your body with nutritious fuel that is convenient for you, take time to acknowledge the One who feeds you, and then get moving in the Kingdom of God—the purpose for which your convenient fuel is given!

Health Lesson:

Today we want to encourage everyone to write down a summary of your experiences over the past week. Reflection is a learning experience, and it's important to acknowledge your progress. You have 1 full week under your belt! Congratulations!! AND you survived…some of you better than others but you are still going strong.

I certainly want every one of you to rave about all of your wins and how much you are enjoying this plan so far! However, there may be some of you out there that don't quite feel the same way…please don't suffer in silence. It is important to acknowledge the things you are struggling with as well. If you're feeling it, there are others out there that probably are too. A former Trainee didn't lose 1 pound the first TWO WEEKS, but ended up losing 14 lbs by the end of the program! So, don't worry about the scale…just keep going!

WHAT TO DO:

STARTING THE SEVEN DAY CLEANSE TODAY. We will add a 7-Day detoxing program to our Getting Healthy regimen. I recommend a cleanse that will detoxify the blood and all the major organs. Do not settle for a cheap substitute that simply empties the colon. This isn't a colonoscopy prep. This is a steady cleansing over one week that should not interrupt your routine in any way except to help you have more energy and get rid of any aches you may be experiencing. Keep eating as you are each day; nothing else changes. Just add the cleanse.

Food Journal - *What I ate today:*

_____

_____

_____

_____

_____

_____

_____

Comments - *How did I feel today & what did I learn?*

_____

_____

_____

_____

_____

_____

_____

_____

What do I need to work on:

_____

_____

_____

_____

_____

_____

_____

Day 20

Read It and Do It!

Therefore whosoever heareth these sayings of mine, and doeth them, I will liken him unto a wise man, which built his house upon a rock: And the rain descended, and the floods came, and the winds blew, and beat upon that house; and it fell not: for it was founded upon a rock. And every one that heareth these sayings of mine, and doeth them not, shall be likened unto a foolish man, which built his house upon the sand: And the rain descended, and the floods came, and the winds blew, and beat upon that house; and it fell: and great was the fall of it. Matthew 7:24-27

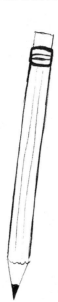

What is the difference between the two builders whose story was the climax of the "Sermon on the Mount?" Both of them were able to build a house. Both had knowledge of construction, and would surely have anticipated that someday adversity would come. One was wise; one was foolish. And Jesus plainly states to his listeners that the wisdom is in the doing. All of us are learning how to improve our health positions. We appreciate the years of research done across the world to improve our lives. We care about our children and our futures. But not all of us will put into practice what we have heard and learned. Your "house" is the temple of the Holy Spirit, and you build up your physical house or tear it down every time you eat. If you are wise in what you do, your house will weather the storms of aging. When your appetites are submitted to God, you are equipped to build on the Rock! Do it!

Health Lesson: Antioxidants Squelch Inflammation

Remember that what you are doing in this program is healing your body at the cellular level. Understanding the function of free radicals and inflammation in your body and how to avoid it will help you move to a higher health position. Here is what *Dr. Deanna's Healing Handbook* says:

When free radicals are on the attack, they don't just kill cells to acquire their missing molecule. "If free radicals simply killed a cell, it wouldn't be so bad... the body could just regenerate another one," he says. "The problem is free radicals often injure the cell, damaging the DNA, which creates the seed for disease." When a cell's DNA changes, the cell becomes mutated. It grows abnormally and reproduces abnormally -- and quickly.

As early as 1992 *TIME* magazine was writing about life at the cellular level and in particular how the chronic disease process works. The "remedy" to fast paced aging is antioxidants – which are vitamins. Dr. Packer in his book, *The Antioxidant Miracle*, says, "A steady regimen of anti-oxidants both on the body and inside the body coupled with lifestyle changes that include an antioxidant rich diet and moderate exercise, is an excellent way to do our part to prevent and protect ourselves from accelerated aging," which again all begins at the cellular level.

Dr. Packer identifies the superhero antioxidants as Vitamin A, C, E, Alpha Lipoic Acid, and CoQ10. If you give the body enough Alpha Lipoic Acid the body will make the glutathione it needs. Glutathione is important to detoxify our bodies at the cellular level. These antioxidant vitamins must all be present and work in concert to get the optimal anti-inflammatory and thus anti-aging effect.

WHAT TO DO:

NO EATING AFTER 7pm during the next month. It isn't always possible, but your daily eating routine should be over by 7pm. The body needs to fast for 12 hours optimally. Two suggestions for you night owls that end up eating a 4th or 5th meal - detox tea and/or GO TO BED. The body detoxes from 10 pm until 2 am and needs to be resting for the greatest detoxing efficiency. The more rest you allow yourselves during the detox, the better results you'll see. Do not be surprised by fatigue or a slight headache, during these first few days. IT WILL GET BETTER!!! You are cleaning up your system.

Stay with your Seven Day Cleanse

Graduating from high school at 289 pounds, my daughter Anna Joy, had given up on being healthy and was considering stomach stapling surgery. Now she is a petite size 10, and an enthusiastic health coach. Read her success story, see pictures, and enjoy her recipes at www.annajoysjourney.wordpress.com

Food Journal - *What I ate today:*

_____

_____

_____

_____

_____

_____

_____

Comments - *How did I feel today & what did I learn?*

_____

_____

_____

_____

_____

_____

_____

_____

What do I need to work on:

_____

_____

_____

_____

_____

_____

_____

Day 21

Don't Faint!

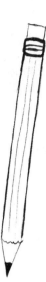

And let us not be weary in well doing: for in due season we shall reap, if we faint not. Galatians 6:9

We are half way through the Appetite for God Program, and the novelty and excitement has been replaced with a certain amount of discipline and perseverance. How often we quote this verse when praying for a loved one or witnessing to a neighbor. This verse declares that the results of doing well are as sure and predictable as a garden that produces food at harvest. Plant the seeds, pull the weeds, and persevere!

Your commitment to health will have its wearying moments. Why not just one bag of greasy flavor-enhanced fries from that old fast-food favorite of yours? Consider that those fries unnaturally spike your blood sugar and douse your gut flora with genetically modified artery clogging oil and set your delicate neurological system buzzing to death with excitotoxins!

In Galatians, that's called fainting, and Paul says, "Don't do it." Hold on to the promise and anticipate the health breakthrough you've always wanted. You are planting the seeds, and God will bless your commitment to be faithful through the growing season!

Health Lesson:

I love the way vegan pea protein satisfies my hunger and fuels me with energy. Protein is the only nutrient that satisfies hunger. Remember your junk food days when you were hungry just an hour after eating? Bread and sugar seesaw your body's balance, and leave you craving more and more and more.

I want to give you an article called "Brains of Children with ADHD Show Protein Deficiency." The research sample is very small, so I don't draw hard and fast conclusions, but it does raise good questions. As long as U.S. research is focused solely on whether a drug works or not, we will not identify the root cause of so much misery that is new with our children's generation. Go to the multimedia section of www.AppetiteforGod.com to read the article.

Your gut bacteria are responsible for producing the essential amino acid, tryptophan, and eating food that has been sprayed with glyphosate, the active ingredient of Roundup, damages gut bacteria's ability to produce this essential amino acid. Here is a summary of current research from *Dr. Deanna's Healing Handbook*:

The presence of glyphosate in the gut inhibits the breakdown of protein into three essential amino acids: phenylalanine, tyrosine, and tryptophan. This breakdown is part of the "shikimate pathway," which is absent in all mammals. For this reason, the manufacturers of gut disrupting herbicides claim that it is safe and nontoxic for humans even though we depend on our gut bacteria for the synthesis of amino acids, and these bacteria are profoundly affected by exposure to herbicides.

Dr. Johansson reported that children with ADHD have a 50 percent lower level of tryptophan, which is important for the production of serotonin, 95% of which is produced in the gut. In addition to depression, serotonin deficiency is associated with greater impulsivity, which is a core symptom of ADHD.

Since the 1990s when herbicides began to be used on food crops engineered to survive their poisonous application, various diseases and conditions have increased dramatically. Scientists are attributing the increase in digestive issues, obesity, autism, Alzheimer's disease, depression, Parkinson's disease, liver disease, cancer, and ADHD to the disruption of the gut biome.

WHAT TO DO:

Are you ready to clean out your pantry again? Read every label. Throw away wheat, corn (including high fructose corn syrup), soy (including lecithin), sugar, and canola/cottonseed/corn oil. That stuff sneaks in there without us thinking about it. It's amazing to think about how much pesticide/herbicide laden food we have eaten since it became so common a decade ago.

All genetically modified food (corn, soy, sugar, canola/cottonseed oil) is artificially designed to survive being sprayed with Roundup. Our gut flora are damaged by glyphosate, the active ingredient that keeps our gut flora from protecting our immunity, our digestion, and our well-being. We must avoid every food grown by genetically modified engineering.

Here is a great To Do list that will keep you going. We are a half way through!

1. Drink lots of water!!

2. Lemon is a natural detoxifier and also alkalizes your water and thus your body. So at home or out, ADD LEMON! You can also carry lemon essential oil with you as well. Squeeze lemon into hot water each morning for a detoxing boost.

3. You can have 1-2 detoxing teas every day, but start with two daily as it will help you flush toxins and negative withdrawal symptoms quickly and gently. Detox tea is great to relax before bed, and it will work while your organs are not distracted with the work of digestion.

4. Designate an hour in the kitchen early each week (or the weekend before) to do all your food 'prep' - chopping veggies, making a batch of protein bars, etc., making dinner time quick & easy throughout the week!

5. The only time you should be stepping on the scale is once a week and I like MONDAY MORNINGS!! Do not obsess with numbers. We don't lose weight to get healthy. We get healthy and then (most of us) naturally lose weight. You will lose inches as well as aches and fatigue. I was especially surprised by clearer thinking. I hadn't really noticed how foggy my brain functioned until it improved with the clean-up!

Food Journal - *What I ate today:*

_____
_____
_____
_____
_____
_____
_____

Comments - *How did I feel today & what did I learn?*

_____
_____
_____
_____
_____
_____
_____
_____

What do I need to work on:

_____
_____
_____
_____
_____
_____

Day 22

Appetite for God: An Example from Africa

Be kindly affectioned one to another with brotherly love; in honor preferring one another; Not slothful in business; fervent in spirit; serving the Lord; Rejoicing in hope; patient in tribulation; continuing instant in prayer; Distributing to the necessity of saints; given to hospitality. Romans 12:10-13

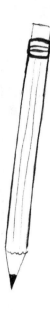

One of the profound ways that I realign my appetites to please God is to visit the beautiful country of Uganda every year, where I am drawn to join my heart with people of incredible faith. I have seen and heard and learned many lessons of significance in Uganda, but all of them seem to fit under this one broad category–I have met a people for whom sustaining life depends on God ALONE. God is all they have, and He is abundantly enough.

People pray for work, and are so grateful for a means of income. They seek after education–to be able to read and write–another supernatural gift that God is giving to thousands through His church. Daily food–when it is there, they are full of gratitude; and when it isn't, the children pray, believing that God would sustain their bodies in health. The food is grown in rich soil in small plots. Surely the health of the people has to do with the quality of farming. Fruits and vegetables are what we would call organic and pay double for. But first, they pray, because not everyone has food every day. God has given them a perspective of food that I want. I need God more than I need food. The Ugandan Christians are living proof.

We were no spring chicken youth group and once or twice I thought about what we would do if somebody had an appendicitis or a heart attack. We would do what the Ugandans do. We would pray in faith, knowing that we have a compassionate Father who heals the sick. His divine intervention is expected and common.

Their homes are built of simple homemade red clay bricks. Paint is far too expensive. Some have concrete floors, some dirt. But all of the Ugandans we met were rich in hospitality. It's interesting that the list Paul gives in Romans 12–the "present your bodies and transform your mind" chapter–are all things that don't require money to accomplish. The Ugandans are incredibly kind, exceedingly honoring of "the visitors," hardworking and fervent in their service to the Lord, full of joy, instant in prayer, full of hospitality–I saw Romans 12 lived out. It is no longer words on a page. It is a group of people who live out their Appetite for God in their day-to-day lives, and hold nothing back in giving to our little group of American adventurers.

What if God was all I had? I mean like a Ugandan–no money, no food, no security, no suburban mansion, no indoor plumbing, no health care. When a tiny bit of our security is diminished, we instinctively respond by hoarding. They have never had it, and because of their great appetite for God who is truly all they have, they give lavishly.

The result is a wildfire of gospel spread. Revival. Hunger for more of God. Joy in sacrifice. Celebration of real life. James writes that God has chosen the poor of this world to be rich in faith. I have spent time with that kind of rich folk. I have a fresh longing to know how to live life with an Appetite for God.

Health Lesson:

The twelve-hour window...

Deep cleansing takes [a night's] time. Imagine your body as a city. Just like a city needs to budget its finances, your body needs to budget its energetic resources. Your daily energy is limited, so your body must constantly prioritize how it gets distributed.

Digestion is one of the most energy-consuming functions of the body (remember last Thanksgiving's food coma?). So if your body is constantly tied up with digestion during the detox, it will put deeper cleansing on hold. Our answer to this: the Twelve-Hour Window. After your evening meal, leave a twelve-hour window before having your morning shake. If you have your evening shake at 7pm, you should have your morning shake at 7am or later.

If you fill up your belly late at night, and eat early again the next day, your body isn't given the opportunity to clean house. The Twelve-Hour Window is challenging to make happen every day, but committing to it will help you get the most out of your Clean Detox. Note: It is okay to have water or herbal tea during the Twelve-Hour Window.

WHAT TO DO:

Although the liver is the body's largest internal cleansing organ, even more cleansing occurs through the skin. Remember, what goes on the skin can be absorbed through the skin via the two circulatory systems, the blood and the lymph, reaching every major organ of the body within seconds. Apply only pure, safe, and beneficial products to your skin.

Read the following article that will help you read the labels and avoid dangerous cosmetic additives on your skin.

Why Pure and Safe Skin Care Makes a Difference for your Family

After eating clean for about a year, I realized that I was still feeding my body toxins, not through my digestion, but through my skin. It's time for another cupboard check, but this time not in your kitchen. Check the bathroom and travel kit for these little known toxins in your soap, shampoo, toothpaste, lotions, and other personal care products.

Parabens

Parabens are an anti-mold preservative found in many skincare products, with the two most common forms, methylparaben and proplyparaben. The chemical structure of a paraben is close to that of estrogen and can fit into estrogen receptors (like docking stations) on cells and this causes a disruption at the cellular level. Constantly sending false estrogenic messages to cells can negatively impact the endocrine system.

In 2004, a study by the University of Reading in the United Kingdom found concentrations of parabens, particularly methylparaben, in human breast tumors. The study examined only the presence of parabens in the tumors but did not determine that they were the cause of the tumors. A follow up study released in 2012 confirmed the presence of parabens in 99% of tested cancerous breast tissue, but did not make a direct connection to the cancer and the parabens.

Phthalates

Phthalates are chemical ingredients that give plastics their elasticity and change the texture and quality of skincare products. As with parabens, phthalates are considered estrogen disruptors and the cause of reproductive problems, especially in males. They also have been indicated as causing fat-related health risks.

A University of Rochester Medical Center study connected common chemicals to rising obesity rates. The analysis found that several phthalate metabolites showed a positive correlation with abdominal obesity. Men with the highest levels of phthalates in their urine had more belly fat and insulin resistance. Researchers adjusted for other factors that could influence the results, such as the men's age, race, food intake, physical activity levels and smoking.

Sulfates

Sulfates generally act as detergents or foaming agents and are found in cleansers and shampoos. Tests show that Sodium Lauryl Sulfate can penetrate into the eyes as well as systemic tissues (brain, heart, liver, etc.) and show long-term retention in those tissues, especially when used in soaps and shampoos.

This is especially important in infants, where considerable growth is occurring and because a much greater uptake occurs in the tissue of younger eyes. SLS also changes the amounts of some proteins in cells in eye tissue of all ages. SLS forms nitrates. When SLS is used in shampoos and cleansers containing nitrogen-based ingredients, it can form carcinogenic nitrates that can enter the blood stream in large numbers. They can cause eye irritations, skin rashes, hair loss, scalp scurf similar to dandruff, and allergic reactions. SLS produces nitrosamines, potent carcinogens that cause the body to absorb nitrates at higher levels than eating nitrate-contaminated food like hot dogs or lunch meat.

Dr. David H. Fine, the chemist who uncovered NDELA contamination in cosmetics, estimates that a person would be applying 50 to 100 micrograms of nitrosamine to the skin each time he or she used a nitrosamine-contaminated cosmetic. By comparison, a person consuming sodium nitrate-preserved bacon is exposed to less than one microgram of nitrosamine. SLS and all its varieties are very harsh detergents that strip the skin's moisture barrier, which is linked to immunity and disruption of skin health, in addition to associated dry, itchy skin. One rule of thumb to remember — if it foams, it may not be your friend.

Petroleum

Commonly used by many skincare companies, petroleum in the form of mineral oil (which has many names) is a cheap medium that can be used as a moisturizing agent and transports other ingredients like fragrance. In many European countries petroleum – mineral oil - is banned as an ingredient in skincare products.

Petroleum can contain known carcinogens (cancer-causing chemicals). Additionally, these products block moisture from escaping the skin, and clog pores. They offer a false sense of hydration, when actually they prevent the action of your skin's natural fats to act to provide a moisture barrier.

Artificial colors and fragrances

Fragrances in lotions, shampoos, and many other cosmetic products are composed of aromatic hydrocarbons. Perfumes and products containing fragrance can contain many hundreds of chemicals to produce a distinct scent. A significant number of these aromas are derived from petroleum. These chemicals have been associated with allergic reactions and hormone disruption. Some fragrance chemicals have not been assessed for safety. Until all fragrance ingredients are disclosed on the label, consumers cannot know what is in a particular fragrance; therefore it's best to avoid synthetic fragrances altogether. Use an essential oil many of which are full of antioxidant support.

Conclusion

"Bargain" cosmetics and personal care products don't just go on our bodies. They go IN our bodies. We understand that our diets have made us sick or healthy, and we need quality meat and fresh vegetables to feed and nourish our bodies. What we put on our skin is also feeding our bodies. If you wouldn't eat a hotdog, why would you let dangerous chemicals reach your joints and brain through your skin?

Head for the cabinet and read the labels!

Food Journal - *What I ate today:*

_____
_____
_____
_____
_____
_____
_____

Comments - *How did I feel today & what did I learn?*

_____
_____
_____
_____
_____
_____
_____
_____

What do I need to work on:

_____
_____
_____
_____
_____
_____
_____

Day 23

The Bread of Life

Labour not for the meat which perisheth, but for that meat which endureth unto everlasting life, which the Son of man shall give unto you: for him hath God the Father sealed. Our fathers did eat manna in the desert; as it is written, He gave them bread from heaven to eat. Then Jesus said unto them, Verily, verily, I say unto you, Moses gave you not that bread from heaven; but my Father giveth you the true bread from heaven. For the bread of God is he which cometh down from heaven, and giveth life unto the world.
John 6:27, 31-33

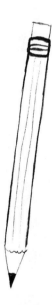

When Jesus miraculously fed thousands of people with a few loaves of barley bread, the people were very willing to follow Him. With Jesus, they would never be hungry, food would always be plentiful, and so many uncertainties of life would be eliminated. So they chased after Him, and greatly relieved at finding Him, they fully expected more. Jesus confronted their motives—they hadn't come to learn about God's kingdom. They came because they ate and were filled (v. 26).

People today still follow Jesus merely for the material blessing they hope to receive. He will get them out of trouble. He will provide what they need. He will make life comfortable. And Jesus still responds, "have you come to Me to understand eternal life, or merely to receive material blessing?"

During this health transformation, we are letting go of tradition, social acceptance, chronic illness and addictions to sugar and processed foods because it is our simple duty. We are choosing not to merely eat and be filled, but rather to fuel our bodies so our minds are the clearest, our energy is the highest, and our health the most promising. Because understanding God's Kingdom is the driving force that moves us to give it all. May the Holy Spirit teach us how to have an Appetite for God that exceeds all other desires in life. Let's trade our focus on manna for a passion for the Bread of Life!

Health Lesson:

Over the next couple weeks, I'm going to highlight the foods on your "AVOID LIST" to give you some background on why they don't serve your bodies. For me, understanding the why behind it helps me shift my mindset from "I can't have that" to "I don't want that". Today, we'll start with the biggest culprit of them all - SUGAR!!!!!!!

Health Issues Related to Sugar Addiction

Sugar has many destructive effects on the human body, including but not limited to, damaging, altering and disrupting proper function of the nervous system, endocrine system, metabolic system, cardiovascular system, gastrointestinal system and immune system as well as primary organs like the liver, kidneys, colon and pancreas.

The list of health problems associated with sugar is enormous and too large to go into completely in one article, but some of the most common include:

- depression
- mood swings
- irritability
- depletion of mineral levels
- hyperactivity
- anxiety or panic attacks
- chromium deficiency
- depletion of the adrenal glands
- type 2 diabetes
- hypoglycemia
- obesity
- Candida overgrowth
- high cholesterol
- anti-social behavior such as that found in crime and delinquency
- anger control issues
- insomnia
- decreased immune function
- aggression
- neurotransmitter deficiencies
- high blood pressure
- heart disease
- asthma
- alcoholism
- acne
- PMS
- OCD
- Fibromyalgia
- attention deficit
- cancer
- binging
- obesity
- chronic fatigue
- addiction
- hormone imbalance

The consumption of sugar is one of the three major causes of degenerative disease in America according to the American Diabetes Association. Sugar is so destructive it can probably be linked to just about any health condition you think of and then some. One of the most important issues for anyone living with a chronic illness is the impact sugar has on the immune system.

Sugar suppresses the immune system. Regardless of whether you're trying to improve your health or protect it, removing sugar from your diet is probably one of the most important things you can do for yourself and your health. If you are under the weather or a child is sick, sugar is especially not good because it depletes the immune system needed for health restoration.

WHAT TO DO:

Check your refrigerator and pantry labels. Get rid of any items that have snuck sugar into your house without you knowing it!

Food Journal - *What I ate today:*

_____

_____

_____

_____

_____

_____

_____

Comments - *How did I feel today & what did I learn?*

_____

_____

_____

_____

_____

_____

_____

_____

What do I need to work on:

_____

_____

_____

_____

_____

_____

_____

Day 24

Measuring Your Appetite

God, who at sundry times and in divers manners spake in time past unto the fathers by the prophets, Hath in these last days spoken unto us by his Son, whom he hath appointed heir of all things, by whom also he made the worlds; Who being the brightness of his glory, and the express image of his person, and upholding all things by the word of his power, when he had by himself purged our sins, sat down on the right hand of the Majesty on high. Hebrews 1:1-3

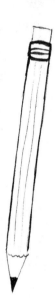

The Hebrew writer begins his book with an entire chapter about Jesus, and it is uncharacteristic and strange to settle in a chapter that doesn't even mention human beings. I want spiritual food that applies to me. My prayers assume to answer the question, what is God going to do for me? I want to thank Him for His goodness to me!

Could I write a chapter, like the Hebrew writer, that doesn't even bother to mention people? His appetite is so fixed on the Savior that his awe and love flow through words of honor and worship. When I meditate on the breathtaking heavenly scenes where angels revere the Savior, I realize that my appetite for worship needs to increase, and my appetite for asking for more needs to decrease.   I know He sends His angels as ministering spirits to lift me out of impossibilities!(v. 14) But the Hebrew writer exhorts me not to focus on the angels and what they do for me. I must fix my eyes on Jesus! He is the Heir of eternity, the Creator of the worlds; by Himself He became the priest forever to purge our sins, and He sits, work finished, as King Jesus at the right hand of God! My prayer today is, Lord, give me an appetite for God!"

For the Lord is a great God, and a great King above all gods. In His hand are the deep places of the earth: the strength of the hills is His also. The sea is His, and He made it: and His hands formed the dry land. O come, let us worship and bow down: let us kneel before the Lord our maker. For He is our God; and we are the people of His pasture, and the sheep of His hand. Psalm 95:3-7

Health Lesson:

Here's the UGLY truth for all of you "diet" and "zero" lovers...and this stuff is not just in sodas - if you see 'light' or 'sugar-free' anything, BE WARNED! READ THE LABEL!! Go to the multimedia section of www.AppetiteforGod.com and read Dr. Mercola's article on Splenda.

By now you can name the four genetically modified food groups without even thinking. You automatically turn the package over to the ingredient list, and instinctively put it back when it says "sugar," or "high fructose corn syrup." Here is a chart that illustrates how recent the genetically modified seed industry has taken over the food supply. Look at chronic disease in young and old, and you will see a skyrocketing correlation between foods altered and nutrition depleted, and the dates in the following chart.

Food	Year GMO Introduced	% of U.S. Crops GMO
Soy	1996	94% in 2011
Cottonseed	1996	90% in 2011
Corn	1996	88% in 2011
Canola Oil	1996	90% in 2010
Papaya	1998	80% in 2010
Alfalfa	2005	(cattle feed only as of 2011)
Sugar Beets	2005	90% as of 2009
Milk	1995	17% of cows injected with rBGH growth hormone as of 2007
Aspartame	1965	Found in over 6,000 products

A Canadian report on the nutritional value of non-GMO corn reported the following:

Non GMO corn contains 437 times more calcium, 56 times more magnesium, and 7 times more manganese. The GMO corn contained high levels of glyphosate and formaldehyde, both toxic to people and animals.

WHAT TO DO:

Treat your family by introducing a new flavor to family dinner tonight. Tumeric has been called the world's healthiest food. Have you ever used it in cooking? Make a salad dressing with walnut oil. Modify a family recipe, replacing sugar and grains with nut flour and stevia. This week we bought organic chicken and cut it up into "nuggets," dipped it in egg, and coated it with coconut flour; then fried it in coconut oil. Too many calories for weight loss, but after two years, I can afford an occasional splurge. Chicken nuggets at the fast food joints always made me and my youngest daughter sick. Now I understand why--they contain more than 30 ingredients and are flavor-enhanced with MSG, and fried in GMO cooking oil. I always have this picture in my mind of holding a gallon of Roundup with the wand stuck in my mouth when I think about eating GMO foods. No thanks.

Food Journal - *What I ate today:*

_____
_____
_____
_____
_____
_____
_____

Comments - *How did I feel today & what did I learn?*

_____
_____
_____
_____
_____
_____
_____
_____

What do I need to work on:

_____
_____
_____
_____
_____
_____
_____
_____

Day 25

Praying Through Weakness

Watch ye and pray, lest ye enter into temptation. The spirit truly is ready, but the flesh is weak. Mark 14:38

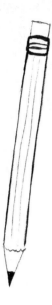

Is the craving for sugar still calling to you? After all you have learned about healing and health, are you still tempted to drive through a fast food window? It always amazes me to talk to people who would rather destroy their bodies over a couple of decades with addictive food laden with chemicals, than to choose health and avoid the chronic illness that is predictably ahead.

I am thankful you have chosen to change your life. You understand that God wants you to walk in health. You will not be mastered by high calorie, nutrition depleted pseudo-food. Even the health and strength of our nation is dependent upon people taking responsibility for their own heath.

The Holy Spirit wants to teach you what it means to pray, "Lead us not into temptation, but deliver us from evil." When your body is longing for sugar and yearning for a hot loaf of fresh bread, it is time for a lesson in prayer. Fix a cup of tea, confess your desires to God, and ask Him to help you to have an Appetite for God that is bigger than the appetite of your flesh. The desires for junk food will not go away overnight. The addiction has been a long time forming. But God expects us to be free and it is our duty as custodians of His temple, our bodies. And His freedom includes surrendering our appetites to His plan and purpose. When you have prayed through to victory, the liberty in Christ will be bigger than anything you have ever experienced.

Health Lesson:

Today is the last day of our seven-day detox cleanse. You have begun the elimination of toxins from your blood and all major organs, and for many of you, weight loss will accelerate, because fat cells are less necessary to store toxins.

Let's address one more way to keep toxins OUT! If you enjoyed a diet coke before this program, I hope you have already eliminated them from your daily routine. I know a couple of teenagers who were addicted to Monster and other energy drinks, who switched to an antioxidant vitamin drink. They have saved their adrenals and so much more.

Aspartame, the artificial sweetener in diet drinks, is the most frequent food additive for adverse reactions reported to the FDA. Nothing is being done about this dangerous chemical. Why not? Monsanto, who owns the patent on most GMO food including Nutrasweet, advises the FDA on its guidelines. Go to the multimedia section of www.AppetiteforGod.com and read Dr. Mercola's article, *"Aspartame: By Far the Most Dangerous Substance Added to Most Foods Today."*

7 Side Effects of Soda

Phosphoric Acid - Weakens bones and rots teeth

Excessive Artificial Sweeteners - Makes you crave more

Caramel Color - Made from chemical caramel, which is purely cosmetic. It doesn't add flavor yet is tainted with carcinogens.

Formaldehyde - Carcinogen, it is not added in soda but when you digest aspartame, it will break down into 2 amino acids and methanol = formic acid + formaldehyde (diet sodas)

High Fructose Corn Syrup - A concentrated form of sugar, fructose derived from corn. It increases body fat, cholesterol and triglycerides and it also makes you hungry.

Potassium Benzoate - Preservative that can be broken down to benzene in your body. Keep your soda in the sun and benzene = carcinogen.

Food Dyes - Impaired brain function, hyperactive behavior, difficult focusing and lack of impulse control.

Information by David Sommers

Drink Diet Soda?
You could have **Aspartame** poisoning!

SYMPTOMS:

Fibromyalgia
Spasms
Shooting Pains
Leg Numbness
Cramps
Vertigo
Dizziness
Headaches

Tinnitus
Joint Pain
Unexplainable Depression
Anxiety Attacks
Slurred Speech
Blurred Vision
Memory Loss
Buzzing in Your Ears

Food Journal - *What I ate today:*

_____

_____

_____

_____

_____

_____

_____

Comments - *How did I feel today & what did I learn?*

_____

_____

_____

_____

_____

_____

_____

_____

What do I need to work on:

_____

_____

_____

_____

_____

_____

_____

_____

Day 26

How God Sees Your Struggle

Furthermore we have had fathers of our flesh which corrected us, and we gave them reverence: shall we not much rather be in subjection unto the Father of spirits, and live? For they verily for a few days chastened us after their own pleasure; but he for our profit, that we might be partakers of his holiness. Hebrews 12:9-10

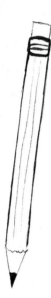

Why do we submit our appetites to God? His discipline is not pleasant, and our flesh still longs to be gratified in unhealthy ways. The Hebrew writer teaches us that we submit our appetites to God in order to live. That's our motive. God disciplines us for our profit, so we can partake of His holiness. That's His motive. How differently we see the experience of discipline!

Take the exodus of the Israelites from Egypt for example. They were suffering from the bitter affliction of slavery. There was groaning under the hardship of Pharaoh's bondage, the endurance of plague after plague, and finally the slaughter of the lamb, and the cries of death among the Egyptians. Then after leaving Egypt, a new set a trials had only begun. From my perspective, the Exodus was a grueling, scary, confusing, and very long journey. The people sinned. Moses became exasperated. God threatened not to go with them. There was hunger, and war, and lots of whining. The parallels in my own life are all too apparent.

Then there is God's perspective. He says in Exodus 19:4, *Ye have seen what I did unto the Egyptians, and how I bare you on eagles' wings, and brought you to Myself.* Wait a minute. Are we talking about the same story? What about the hunger and thirst and the desert and the giants?

That verse gives me a whole new perspective on accepting discipline in my life in order to honor God. Today I want to submit my appetites to God because His pure motive for taking away, and saying no, is my profit, my health, and my holiness. I'm like the children of Israel leaving Egypt seeing only how hard it is to make all these drastic changes. And God sees the very same process as lifting me up on eagles' wings. He carries us through hardship. He delivers us in spite of our whining. And He brings us to a land flowing with milk and honey, though we are too focused on the pain of discipline to figure out that God is bearing us up on eagles' wings every step of the way.

As you submit your appetite to God, ask Him to open your eyes to see the eagles, and your ears to hear His calling. We will endure His discipline together, and the trials will seem lighter because we remind each other of the prize ahead. There is no greater reward than to share in His holiness.

Health Lesson:

If you don't take out the trash at your house, it will pile up, attract pests, and quickly become a problem. Right? During a detox your body takes out its "trash" by eliminating toxins through pores, breathing, kidneys, and the bowels, but daily bowel movements help make sure toxins are not re-absorbed into your system.

Bowel movements can increase when doing the detox. At other times you may be constipated. If you are constipated here are a few ways to resolve it:

1. Add a scoop of fiber to your diet twice a day. You know you are using too much if gas and bloating occurs. Adjust your fiber intake to aid your liver and maximize the cleanliness of your gut. Each person will be different.

2. Stay hydrated: Drink enough water so you use the bathroom once every hour or so.

3. Eat fiber-rich foods: Include leafy green salad, cherries, figs, prunes, pears, aloe juice, warm lemon water, or green vegetable juices.

4. Move it: Do some movement and exercise. Walking and light aerobics work great.

5. Use a natural magnesium citrate supplement to help restore healthy magnesium levels and increases calcium intake to encourage natural stress relief and healthy bowel movements. Vitamin C as Ascorbic Acid can also assist moving your bowels. Purchase these at your local natural food store.

WHAT TO DO:

Prepare a very warm bath and add ½ cup baking soda or a bottle of peroxide, and soak until the water cools. You are aiding your skin to detox. Your liver can't do it all!

Food Journal - *What I ate today:*

_____

_____

_____

_____

_____

_____

_____

_____

Comments - *How did I feel today & what did I learn?*

_____

_____

_____

_____

_____

_____

_____

_____

What do I need to work on:

_____

_____

_____

_____

_____

_____

_____

_____

Day 27

Comfort Food and Grieving People

Whose end is destruction, whose god is their belly. Philippians 3:19

Give no offense in anything, that the ministry be not blamed. II Corinthians 6:3

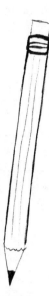

Fox News recently reprinted an excoriating rebuke to pastors and churches that made our church staff physician's no-nonsense exhortations to get healthy seem warm and fuzzy. Dr. Scott Stoll minces no words, declaring that fundamental Christians are by far the heaviest of all religious groups.

The lead researcher observed, "America is becoming a nation of gluttony and obesity and churches are a feeding ground for this problem." According to a Northwestern University study, people who attend church or Bible study once a week are 50% more likely to be obese. Worse yet, another study found that the clergy were 76% overweight, compared to 61% of the general population.

I don't really want to think about this, much less talk about it, because I have lived my life in appreciation of the comfort value of chocolate. Grieving people too often salve their pain with food not realizing that refined and processed foods are as addictive as cocaine, and are a root cause of depression only compounding their pain. And in the middle of the church, there is no incentive to examine ourselves because in our hearts we're acting like Gnostics—the physical body is corrupt and of no consequence, and we'll just work to be more spiritual.

In the last two years, I had some health scares. My doctor told me I had a large abdominal tumor, and I needed to update my Last Will and Testament before seeing a specialist. I was lethargic because of arthritic pain in my joints. It hurt to move at 58 years old! There were also "spots" on my liver that "needed to be watched." My skin when wounded did not heal quickly; my memory dropped details that used to come effortlessly. My immune system did not fight off multiple bouts of shingles. To use my pastor Dr. Parish's words, I was "sick and tired, and sick and tired of being sick and tired."

Several months ago, my life changed radically. My daughter found a health and wellness program that she dragged me into, along with her sisters and their families. We have collectively lost over 250 pounds since. Now, as Christians, we are at the phase of reflecting on what in the world happened to us, and why we didn't figure it out years ago!

I realize now I ate for comfort, and for relief from grief after being widowed three times. Amid the earth quaking changes, we rebuilt family togetherness around food which we now understand was destroying our health. We were bonding around our "appetites" and that got quickly out of control. We struggled to simply meet the demands of work and family with little energy leftover to think about God's kingdom on earth where our children and grandchildren will grow up.

I'm so amazingly grateful for what has happened to us, I have to invite you to get in on it. I want my son to take me elk hunting in Alaska for my 80th birthday, and maybe you should plan to come too. I want to talk to you about taking control of your own health. I am passionate about being healthy! Today, my divinely designed body has no arthritis, no tumors, no foggy thinking, no aches and pains, and I've lost 35 pounds.

My beautiful teenage daughter who wore a size 22 to her senior prom only a year later dresses for success in a stunning size 10. It cost me no effort and no money—seriously! It was easy, there were no monster exercise routines, and we are saving time and money with the new lifestyle! I said, "no effort and no money," but I didn't say "no sacrifice."

I had to give up my gluttonous addictions to foods that were hurting me. I chose health instead of diabetes, heart disease, hypertension, and arthritis, and I want to encourage you to make that choice too.

Finally, I'm embarrassed by the article in Fox News. We, the Church, are being indicted and shamed by the World for our appetites. I have brought reproach upon the church by my neglect and the media is calling us on the carpet. It gets a little lonely out here living life where food is not at the center of what we do. I want you to join me, so I am telling you how we changed our routine to get fit for God's kingdom work. It has become more than physical maintenance; it's also spiritual for me. If we as the body of Christ would honor God with our physical bodies, the world would sit up and take notice (Exodus 15:26).

Health Lesson:

Whether you agree with him or not, you need to read this scathing article from Fox News about the state of the church. It truly motivated me to think about what my non-church going friends think about the institutions of faith that are measurably taken over by the sin of gluttony! Go to the multimedia section of www.AppetiteforGod.com and read "Fat in Church" by Scott Stoll, MD.

WHAT TO DO:

Make the commitment to reject all food addictions. The next time your church or civic group has a "potluck" dinner, take a healthy living foods dish that tastes good. Drink a protein shake before you go so you won't be tempted by that GMO sugar laden table of pseudo-food called dessert! Give a gentle but joyful answer to all those folks who are going to start asking, "What happened to you!"

Food Journal - *What I ate today:*

_____

_____

_____

_____

_____

_____

_____

_____

Comments - *How did I feel today & what did I learn?*

_____

_____

_____

_____

_____

_____

_____

_____

What do I need to work on:

_____

_____

_____

_____

_____

_____

_____

Day 28

The Power of a Godly Example

Take, my brethren, the prophets, who have spoken in the name of the Lord, for an example of suffering affliction and of patience. Behold, we count them happy which endure. James 5:10-11

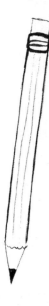

Some of you have changed enough in the last two weeks that people are beginning to take notice. You have lost weight. You have more energy. You are smiling more. Your endurance is beginning to shine through in happiness! Leaders are goal setters. They change their personal lives for the better. They step out of the herd that is mindlessly moving in the wrong direction. James ends his book by reminding us that there is power in setting the example. You are an example too. You have made a decision to submit your appetites to God and reject an immediate focus and goal of feeling good by changing your outward circumstances. You have believed God with your whole heart that you can live with unmet needs and still experience the full joy of the Lord.

Just suppose for a moment that we took James seriously and considered the prophets as our examples. Jeremiah declared, *Before me continually is grief and wounds* (Jeremiah 6:7). Out of his weeping for a nation that hated him comes great assurance—*Call unto me, and I will answer thee, and show thee great and mighty things, which thou knowest not* (Jeremiah 33:3). We all know the promise from Jeremiah's Lamentation, *It is of the LORD's mercies that we are not consumed, because his compassions fail not. They are new every morning: great is thy faithfulness* (Lamentations 3:22-23). But the context of that promise in the preceding twenty verses is gut wrenching horror. How could Jeremiah speak such immortal words out of a place so consumed with hardship?

Jeremiah understood how to walk with his God who loved and cared for him in an upside down world. I love his words from Jeremiah 31:3, *The Lord hath appeared of old unto me, saying, Yea, I have loved thee with an everlasting love: therefore with loving-kindness have I drawn thee.*

Jeremiah knew such deep love from his God in the midst of war and destruction all around him. He heard God calling him as a child—*Before I formed you in the womb, I knew you* (Jeremiah 1:5), and he never stopped listening and obeying. He believed God's promise, *And ye shall seek me, and find me, when ye shall search for me with all your heart* (Jeremiah 29:13), though the promise seemed impossible in his circumstances.

I hear God calling us too. He tells us His great and precious promises are ours if we are willing to take for our example the prophets. Satan will tell you that you are alone. There is no hope. You will never be able to eat or think or sleep normally again. These are LIES. Let's walk as the prophets of old, and find true health by putting our full trust in the One who "knows the plans he has for us." If Jeremiah could speak of everlasting love, and hope, and great faithfulness in his upside down life, we will too!

Health Lesson:

Here in Louisville, Kentucky, we have several healthy restaurant options. Two more upscale restaurants I recommend are the Mayan Café, and Mitchell's Fish Market. Two budget restaurants you can visit are the Chipotle Mexican Grill and Shiraz Mediterranean. Two delicious salad bars (if you ask the server will bring you olive oil, lemon and salt to dress your salads) can be found at Ruby Tuesdays, and Jason's Deli, both chain restaurants found in other cities as well.

I know this is repetitive, but, stay away from sugary oily GM laden dressings! Ask if the seasonings used in the restaurant are free of MSG. Americans eat out an average of 4-5 times a week and for those taking control of their foods it will be difficult to eat out. Food can no longer be entertainment or the driving social force in our lives. Remember food is fuel for a healthy body. It will not have control of us!

When you eat out, don't be afraid to ask for modifications when you order...no cheese, no bread, lemons on the side for dressing, etc. Lots of restaurants are offering gluten-free options these days, so check for that and then modify as best you can. There's actually an app/website called findmeglutenfree.com.

When your friends want to dine out, suggest a healthy option. You'll be surprised how often they are pleasantly surprised by good, clean food!

WHAT TO DO:

Eat out this week and write in your food journal about it. Can you honor your food fitness commitment at the restaurant you chose? DO NOT CHEAT! You've come too far, and you'll be surprised to find yourself feeling sick if you revert to toxic sugar and wheat all of a sudden after weeks of cleaning that junk out of your system!

Food Journal - *What I ate today:*

_____
_____
_____
_____
_____
_____
_____

Comments - *How did I feel today & what did I learn?*

_____
_____
_____
_____
_____
_____
_____

What do I need to work on:

_____
_____
_____
_____
_____
_____
_____

Day 29

The Covenant of Health

And said, If thou wilt diligently hearken to the voice of the LORD thy God, and wilt do that which is right in his sight, and wilt give ear to his commandments, and keep all his statutes, I will put none of these diseases upon thee, which I have brought upon the Egyptians: for I am the LORD that healeth thee. Exodus 15:26

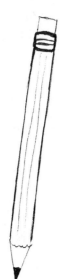

I have witnessed and experienced God's merciful intervention in my life and the lives of my children when I asked Him for healing. God is a giver. His care for us flows from a heart of compassion and mercy. He is the Lord that heals us, the same Lord who healed the children of Israel.

But our healing also has an essential principle that God showed to Israel from the beginning. It is His principle of sowing and reaping. We are commanded to keep all his statutes, and to love His laws. His covenant of mercy is not without responsibility to keep His commandments, statutes and judgments. And so, as the children of Israel obeyed God, they experienced a divine level of health that other nations around them noticed. It was God's blessing, and it was their obedience. They had "none of these diseases." They were blessed with children, and their livestock had healthy offspring, and they were given health above all people.

Therefore it shall come to pass, if ye hearken to these judgments, and keep, and do them, that the LORD thy God shall keep unto thee the covenant and the mercy which he sware unto thy fathers: And he will love thee, and bless thee, and multiply thee: he will also bless the fruit of thy womb, and the fruit of thy land, thy corn, and thy wine, and thine oil, the increase of thy kine, and the flocks of thy sheep, in the land which he sware unto thy fathers to give thee. Thou shalt be blessed above all people: there shall not be male or female barren among you, or among your cattle. And the LORD will take away from thee all sickness, and will put none of the evil diseases of Egypt, which thou knowest, upon thee; but will lay them upon all them that hate thee. Deuteronomy 7:12-15

I think we are afraid to talk much about this, because it is no longer true of the children of God. The church is fat and sick. We don't want people who are precious in God's sight to suffer or feel ashamed. It is arrogant and cruel to blame barrenness or sickness upon an individual who is already in pain. But on the other hand, wouldn't it be sad if the only generation of God's people who were known for their divine health were ones who didn't have the grace of Jesus, who wandered in the wilderness, and who understood so little of God's covenant. We will never point a finger at anyone to show what God has NOT done. His promises are true, and we long to see them fulfilled completely in our day to day living. Let us consider God's plan for us to walk in divine health. Let us seek His guidance and understand his commandments for submitting our appetites to Him. If we fulfilled our part in complete obedience to His natural laws of health, perhaps the church could be known once again as the people who walk in divine health. Because God is still the giver. He is still full of compassion and mercy, and loves to provide all things for His children. There will always be mystery in explaining God's providence and will. He asks us to pray that His will would be done on earth as it is in heaven. In heaven, His will is NO sickness, a garden that is abundantly productive, and no sorrow, not even a sigh. I pray that we will so clearly understand His will for us regarding our food that He can give us all the health He wants to give. We will sow in submission and obedience. We can trust Him to provide the abundant harvest.

Health Lesson:

How to Restore a Healthy Gut

Antibiotics kill both good and bad bacteria in the gut, and their overuse has led to problems such as allergic reactions, resistant bacteria such as MRSA, and permanent damage to the gut flora which control 80 percent of our immunity. Antibiotic use can also result in yeast overgrowth because of the imbalance of your gut bacteria. Symptoms such as athlete's foot, ringworm, or abnormal nail growth may indicate a yeast/fungal infection and a compromised gut.

Replenish your gut flora with the three major strains of live cultures of beneficial bacteria. *Bifidobacteria* and *lactobacillus*, which are beneficial probiotics in our guts, produce antifungal and antibacterial substances that balance the gut flora as well as manufacture B vitamins. You will find *saccharomyces* as a major ingredient in immunity boosters and other probiotic supplements, which is an important beneficial yeast that prevents overgrowth of potentially harmful yeast such as Candida. Candida requires sugar in order to grow; and the Western high-sugar diet is a predisposing factor for the epidemic of candidiasis.

People always ask me if they can just eat yogurt to improve their gut health. Well, here's a troubling fact for you. Commercial flavored yogurt contains 100% more sugar than Lucky Charms cereal. Yogurt is heated to a temperature that kills live cultures, and requires preservatives to increase its grocery store shelf life. So the short answer is no, don't buy yogurt. Make it yourself from raw goat's milk. Sugar free, live culture, fermented food is very good for you.

WHAT TO DO:

How about a movie?

We don't advocate here for not eating meat, but you may want to watch Forks Over Knives, a documentary about the state of health and disease in the US and how people – through dietary changes – have restored their bodies from food related chronic diseases. It is available on Netflix and will probably make some of you feel a lot better about what we're doing. This may be what pushes you to continue the changes even after the 40 days. Remember it's about training ourselves to make better choices. It shouldn't be "I can't have that!" BUT "I don't want that!"

Food Journal - *What I ate today:*

_____

_____

_____

_____

_____

_____

_____

Comments - *How did I feel today & what did I learn?*

_____

_____

_____

_____

_____

_____

_____

_____

What do I need to work on:

_____

_____

_____

_____

_____

_____

_____

_____

Day 30

Health for the Whole Family

And I looked, and rose up, and said unto the nobles, and to the rulers, and to the rest of the people, Be not ye afraid of them: remember the LORD, which is great and terrible, and fight for your brethren, your sons, and your daughters, your wives, and your houses. Nehemiah 4:14

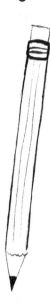

By now you have realized how important it is for everyone in the family to choose health together. This isn't a "diet" where one person abstains from unhealthy food for a few weeks. This program is designed for families to submit their appetites to God to achieve permanent health in service to God. In the Old Testament, there was a wall to restore which required the people to do work they had not done before. Nehemiah was incredibly wise. He gathered people in families to do the work together. He ignored problems he didn't need to address. He would agree with me when I say, "do your best and let the loose ends drag."

I am curious about a man named Shallum. Evidently he didn't have sons, but he was assigned a section of the wall to build, and he completed the work with his daughters! (Nehemiah 3:12) My girls and I have built some walls together, and one of those walls is a wall of health. When the Sanballats and Tobiahs of the world told me my children would never come around, I did what Nehemiah did—I gave them none of my time to listen. I just love Nehemiah.

God is great and awesome, just like Nehemiah said, and the ones we love are so worth fighting for. Let's teach our families how to have permanent health! When Satan clutters your mind with doubt and confusion, respond with the promise of our great and awesome Savior. Here is a truth that calls me to submit my appetites to God today—

He that sows to the Spirit shall of the Spirit reap life everlasting. And let us not be weary in well doing: for in due season we shall reap, if we faint not. As we have therefore opportunity, let us do good unto all men, especially unto them who are of the household of faith. Galatians 6:8-10.

Health Lesson:

FOOD CRAVING defined: An intense desire to consume a specific food, stronger than simply normal hunger.

There is no single explanation for food cravings and can range from the following:

1. Foods that are high in fats, carbohydrates and glucose (chocolate, sweets) affect the brain centers for appetite to produce endorphins and interactions with the opioid system in the brain triggering an addictive effect to occur.

    The consumer of the glucose feels the urge to consume more glucose, much like an alcoholic, because the brain has become conditioned to release "happy hormones" every time glucose is present. This essentially means that the brain physically changes when it becomes used to consuming a mass quantity of a certain chemical, so that the brain can release the highest quantity of "happy hormones" as possible. ("Emotional Eaters" are not really emotional eaters. It is your brain telling you it wants HAPPY HORMONES).

2. When we consume foods that are not CLEAN (providing nutrients and fuel) for the body...the body remains "unsatisfied" creating a craving for the "fuel" that is still needed, even after eating sometimes a large amount of "food". What these statements say to me is that craving for food is a true physical response from your body and it is affecting how you eat. You are not "mental"! I hope this will help people that are not happy with their health and/or body image. Stop "beating yourself up" thinking that you are just "weak" with food mentally! It is a true physical response you are having. This does not release you from the responsibility to do something about your health, but you can give yourself grace and start taking steps to making healthier choices for life when you understand this fact!

You have now been empowered to start taking steps in changing the physical response you might be having to food. Every day that you eat clean and stick to the *Appetite for God* plan, you are making the choice to change! You will retrain your brain to crave the healthy foods with the better choices you make and your body realizes it feels so good when you do! With long-term permanent, healthy eating you will enjoy a life full of energy, health and vitality!

WHAT TO DO:

Boost your brain by walking today. The problem with loss of brain function is there are no symptoms until the problem is massive. We have so much more brain than we need, we forget how critical it is to maintain neurological health. In Dr. Perlmutter's *Better Brain Book*, he recommends CoQ10, Vitamin E, Alpha Lipoic Acid, Vitamin D, and Omega 3's to boost brain health. The protein supplement I have each day along with high quality absorbable nutrition supplements help keep my brain fueled and healthy! Add Dr. Perlmutter's suggestions to your daily regimen, and check out his Facebook page.

SUGAR ADDICTION:
The Perpetual Cycle

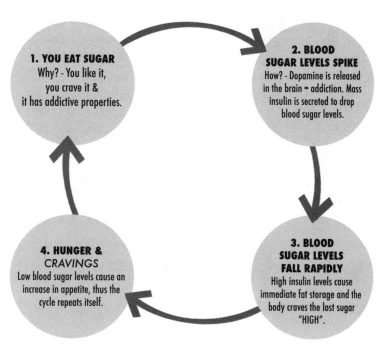

1. YOU EAT SUGAR
Why? - You like it, you crave it & it has addictive properties.

2. BLOOD SUGAR LEVELS SPIKE
How? - Dopamine is released in the brain = addiction. Mass insulin is secreted to drop blood sugar levels.

3. BLOOD SUGAR LEVELS FALL RAPIDLY
High insulin levels cause immediate fat storage and the body craves the lost sugar "HIGH".

4. HUNGER & CRAVINGS
Low blood sugar levels cause an increase in appetite, thus the cycle repeats itself.

Food Journal - *What I ate today:*

_____
_____
_____
_____
_____
_____
_____

Comments - *How did I feel today & what did I learn?*

_____
_____
_____
_____
_____
_____
_____
_____

What do I need to work on:

_____
_____
_____
_____
_____
_____
_____

Day 31

Freedom From Unbridled Appetites

Looking diligently lest any man fail of the grace of God; lest any root of bitterness springing up trouble you, and thereby many be defiled; Lest there be any fornicator, or profane person, as Esau, who for one morsel of meat sold his birthright. Hebrews 12:15-16

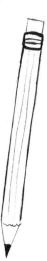

The Hebrew writer is warning us to look diligently to God's grace, the anecdote for the bondage of misusing food and sex. Just as in Acts 15 where Peter warned that controlling the appetite for food and sex are foundational principles for following Christ, the Hebrew writer gives the same warning. When addressing food's pitfalls, he gives us an example, the one who is only known for his surrender of the birthright for a single meal.

The birthright gave the eldest son incredible lifelong privileges including rights to the priesthood and a double portion of inheritance. He would be the head of the family, the patriarch, for life, and would convey special blessings to the next generation. All of this Esau gave up for a single serving of food.

We don't have such dramatic examples in our culture, although many great leaders have surrendered their integrity and credibility in fornication. The surrender to gluttony is more gradual, but as we are warned, its stronghold is just as dangerous and unholy. May God help us as Peter warned, to look diligently to God for grace to remain pure in all areas pertaining to our appetites for food and sex.

Health Lesson:

We have included in the appendix a summary of research on childhood diseases that have skyrocketed in the last decade. In 1976, one in 30 children was learning disabled. Today it is one in 6. In 1980, one child in 27 had asthma. Today it is one in 9. In 1990, one child in 555 developed autism. Today it is one in 50. In examining the worldwide research on what is happening to our children, we found around twenty risk factors that correlated with dramatically decreasing health in kids. One of those risks which is receiving wide publicity and propaganda today is the issue of vaccines. The National Vaccine Information Center publishes research on the risk of vaccines which now total a mind boggling 69 doses by age 18. A medical doctor in England has spent her life treating children with autism, and here is her expert advice to parents who must protect their children's health.

Vaccines may not represent a single cause, but rather "the last straw" which deepens damage already done to the immune system, and causes symptoms to appear. McBride proposes that the "vaccinate every child" rule must be changed and only after a comprehensive health history is obtained on the baby and a urine and stool analysis is done to determine the risk of gut dysbiosis and the baby's immune status. Here are her recommendations:

1. Vaccines for healthy infants with healthy parents and whose tests show normal immune development, given in single vaccines only. A child doesn't get three childhood diseases at once in the environment. The immune system should not be overloaded artificially with multiple vaccines at once.

2. Delayed vaccines when the mother is healthy, but baby shows abnormalities in the immune system, such as allergies, frequent ear infections, or exposure to antibiotics. The child could be retested every six to eight months and vaccinated with single vaccines only when they are ready, and at least six weeks apart.

3. No vaccines for an infant born to a mother with allergic, autoimmune, neurological, or digestive problems. An infant with eczema, asthma, digestive problems or any disorder suggesting a compromised immune system cannot recover from vaccines. Avoid also in younger siblings of children with asthma, allergies, ADHD, epilepsy, and insulin dependent diabetes.

WHAT TO DO:

The Rachel Ray Show hosted a diet book author, whose advice was this-- If you could do just ONE thing for your health to really make a difference, it would be to start your day with a VEGAN PROTEIN SHAKE!! (Making sure you avoid soy and whey) Look for protein sources such as peas, cranberries, and brown rice. Do not use coconut milk as she does in the video if your goal is weight loss. Coconut milk is delicious, but is calorie dense. As you have found out already, the protein and berry shakes are delicious with water!

Go to multimedia section of the www.AppetiteforGod.com website to watch this 4 minute clip that will encourage you to keep doing what you are already doing! The clip is entitled, "The Virgin Diet by Rachel Ray."

Food Journal - *What I ate today:*

_____
_____
_____
_____
_____
_____
_____

Comments - *How did I feel today & what did I learn?*

_____
_____
_____
_____
_____
_____
_____
_____
_____

What do I need to work on:

_____
_____
_____
_____
_____
_____
_____
_____

Day 32

Get Your Belly Full

In the last day, that great day of the feast, Jesus stood and cried, saying, If any man thirst, let him come unto me, and drink. He that believeth on me, as the scripture hath said, out of his belly shall flow rivers of living water. (But this spake he of the Spirit, which they that believe on him should receive...). John 7:37-39

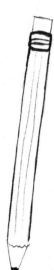

Jesus took the occasion of a feast to explain how the people could really satisfy that hunger and thirst in their bellies. It's a holiday party. People have come expecting to eat until they are full and content. But when their appetite for food is satisfied, a longing remains.

The same is true in our lives when we are so focused on the satisfaction of eating. Our appetite for the Holy Spirit is faint. We feast our way into fatness and ill health, and the emptiness remains.

Then Jesus stands up and cries out to my heart, "satisfy your hunger and thirst with living water! Do I dare believe that there is more than mere food for the body? Could I manage a family, and keep my finances in order, and give to God the burden of provision that consumes my thoughts and desires? What if my energy dries up? What if my bills don't get paid? What if I become flat and boring? What if...? I've forgotten about the uncontrollable expansive grand river whose limitless satisfaction is mine for the asking. I only have to reorder my appetites, and receive!

I am awakening my spiritual appetite. Jesus called out His promise on that feast day to all that believe. I will dare to respond and take my thirst to the One who promises rivers of living water. I don't have to ration the water—the mighty river will provide for all of my appetites, and never decrease its volume. I will drink until His living water flows out of my belly and reaches others with hope and health. The river that carries heavy barges, speed boats and dozing fishermen, which provides water for our entire city and never dries up, is only a miniature illustration of the immense river in the spiritual realm that provides for all who are thirsty for God.

Health Lesson:

Another Detox Tip from Dr Oz: snack mindfully or not at all!

Before you joined the *Appetite for God* program, you may have started innocently snacking on cookies or chips and then realized twenty minutes later that you ate the whole bag. To make matters worse, you weren't even hungry. We've all been there; I have many times in fact. Rather than calling on your own personal guilt monster, give this a thought:

The repeated desire to snack is really a desire to change how we're feeling in the moment. The more we're not conscious of why we're snacking, the more this habit can numb how we really feel. Food can be used for comfort, to relieve boredom, for social connection, or to medicate depression. When these issues arise, recognize them as a call to increase our appetite for God, not our appetite for food! We understand that for some, snacking is helpful in maintaining good energy levels and mood. But before you start grabbing snacks, even if they are clean, check in with yourself and make sure what you're feeling is true hunger. Sometimes finding the right amount to eat everyday takes a little personal experimentation. If you find that you are consistently hungry throughout the day, add a between meal snack of 10 almonds or a protein bar made from your protein powder, because you know the ingredients.

Remember, only protein will satisfy your hunger, so make your snacks pure protein. Never use simple carbs as a snack, such as bread or chips, as these will actually increase your hunger.

WHAT TO DO:

Let's plan a grocery trip to shop for clean foods to provide one meal per day for this week. You can choose a couple of Anna Joy's main dish recipes in the back of the book, and go back to the Getting Started Instructions for suggestions of vegetables and salad fixings. Have you noticed how affordable it is to eat clean after all?

If you are hosting a dinner why not surprise your guests with homemade salad dressing or serve a raw vegetable tray with an avocado dip? There are 6 healthy dressing/dip recipes in the recipe section for you.

TIME TO WEIGH IN! Take and record your weight and measurements again using the chart on page 154. We are getting close to the end, keep up the good work!

Food Journal - *What I ate today:*

_____
_____
_____
_____
_____
_____
_____

Comments - *How did I feel today & what did I learn?*

_____
_____
_____
_____
_____
_____
_____
_____
_____

What do I need to work on:

_____
_____
_____
_____
_____
_____
_____
_____

Day 33

Fasting

Then I proclaimed a fast there, at the river of Ahava, that we might afflict ourselves before our God, to seek of him a right way for us, and for our little ones, and for all our substance. Ezra 8:21

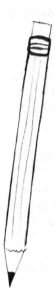

Ezra is leading the people who have spent their lives in captivity in Babylon, greatly influenced by the culture around them. Their children were born there, and had no first hand memory of worshipping the One True God. Ezra stopped to humble himself and to seek God. They needed Him, and more than that, they needed to know their need of Him, and the right way He had planned for each generation. It was a pivotal point of turning in each family. It was time to fast.

Throughout scripture, fasting has been associated with humbling ourselves before God. It refocuses our appetites away from food, and intensifies our seeking of that which is greater than food—

For the kingdom of God is not meat and drink; but righteousness, and peace, and joy in the Holy Ghost. Romans 14:17

Though the specifics of fasting are not commanded, Jesus acknowledged that His followers would fast after He returned to Heaven.

And Jesus said unto them, Can the children of the bridechamber mourn, as long as thebridegroom is with them? but the days will come, when the bridegroom shall be taken from them, and then shall they fast. Matthew 9:15

And throughout history, great leaders have called the church to humble themselves and seek God's direction through fasting. St. Chrysostom wrote to the priests,

Sharpen thy sickle, which thou hast blunted through gluttony—sharpen it by fasting. Lay hold of the pathway which leads towards heaven . . . And how mayest thou be able to do these things? By subduing thy body, and bringing it into subjection. For when the way grows narrow, the corpulence that comes of gluttony is a great hindrance.

John Calvin, in the 16th century said:

Let us say something about fasting, because many, for want of knowing its usefulness, undervalue its necessity, and some reject it as almost superfluous; while, on the other hand where the use of it is not well understood, it easily degenerates into superstition. Holy and legitimate fasting is directed to three ends; for we practice it either as a restraint on the flesh, to preserve it from licentiousness, or as a preparation for prayers and pious meditations, or as a testimony of our humiliation in the presence of God when we are desirous of confessing our guilt before him (Institutes, IV. 12, 14, 15).

Martin Luther wrote:

Of fasting I say this: It is right to fast frequently in order to subdue and control the body. For when the stomach is full, the body does not serve for preaching, for praying, or studying, or for doing anything else that is good. Under such circumstances God's Word cannot remain. But one should not fast with a view to meriting something by it as by a good work.

And John Wesley adds,

Every wise man will refrain his soul, and keep it low; will wean it more and more from all those indulgences of the inferior appetites, which naturally tend to chain it down to earth, and to pollute as well as debase it. Here is another perpetual reason for fasting; to remove the food of lust and sensuality, to withdraw the incentives of foolish and hurtful desires, of vile and vain affections.

A call to fasting and prayer used to be a regular responsibility of American Presidents. President Lincoln made the following proclamation on April 30, 1863:

Whereas, the Senate of the United States, devoutly recognizing the Supreme Authority and just Government of Almighty God, in all the affairs of men and of nations, has, by a resolution, requested the President to designate and set apart a day for National prayer and humiliation.

And whereas it is the duty of nations as well as of men, to own their dependence upon the overruling power of God, to confess their sins and transgressions, in humble sorrow, yet with assured hope that genuine repentance will lead to mercy and pardon; and to recognize the sublime truth, announced in the Holy Scriptures and proven by all history, that those nations only are blessed whose God is the Lord....

Now, therefore, in compliance with the request, and fully concurring in the views of the Senate, I do, by this my proclamation, designate and set apart Thursday, the 30th. day of April, 1863, as a day of national humiliation, fasting and prayer. And I do hereby request all the People to abstain, on that day, from their ordinary secular pursuits, and to unite, at their several places of public worship and their respective homes, in keeping the day holy to the Lord, and devoted to the humble discharge of the religious duties proper to that solemn occasion.

As we make fundamental changes in the ways we fuel our bodies, we are much like Ezra, seeking what his current generation could not know or understand because they had been captive so long. Once we have humbled our minds and bodies by setting aside the appetite for food to see a greater appetite for God, we will discover that there are physical benefits to fasting as well as spiritual. While fasting drives us to seek God for a spiritual breakthrough, the fast is working at the cellular level for a breakthrough from sugar and carb overload to a healthier physical plane of stability and function.

Health Lesson:

We are approaching the last week of our 40 Day health transformation. You should feel much more in control of your hunger and overall health as cravings have subsided and fueling your body has become more routine. IF you want to stretch a bit more, I have something for you to think about again—the health benefits of fasting. If you don't want to think about it, just skip to the WHAT TO DO section. Here is an excerpt from *Dr. Deanna's Healing Handbook*—

Research studies over the past decade suggest that intermittent fasting could reduce the risk of cancer, guard against diabetes and heart disease, help control asthma, and improve brain function while protecting against Parkinson's disease and dementia. A fast starts 10 to 12 hours after the last meal when all of the available glucose in the blood is used up, and the liver begins to convert glycogen and fat to usable energy. The liver produces ketones in the process, which can be used by the brain for fuel. At the Longevity Institute at the University of Southern California, short-term fasts were found to slow the growth of five of eight cancer tumors in animals. Dr. Stephen Freedland of Duke University claims that "under-nutrition without malnutrition" is the only experimental approach that improves survival in animals with cancer.

A 24 hour once-a-month water only fast will raise the level of human growth hormone, which triggers the breakdown of fat, and reduces insulin levels. According to *The American Journal of Cardiology*, this reduces the risk of diabetes and coronary heart disease. Human Growth Hormone is also elevated in other fasting plans, such as limiting your eating to an eight hour window each day (Dr. Mercola recommends 11:00 a.m. to 7:00 p.m.), or the "5:2" fasting plan where two days a week you eat a single meal of less than 600 calories.

Mark Mattson of the NIH Institute on Aging recommends alternate day fasting, where you eat a single meal under 600 calories every other day. He found that after a few weeks, asthma symptoms improved, and inflammation markers decreased. He found that fasting increases brain activity, and boosts the production of a brain protein called brain-derived neurotropic factor by 50 to 400 percent. This protein stimulates the generation of new brain cells and plays a role in learning and memory. It protects brain cells from changes associated with Alzheimer's and Parkinson's. He also found a reduction in insulin resistance.

WHAT TO DO:

Congratulations for successfully completing another week! Some of you aren't seeing the change you wanted and please know that this takes time and we all respond differently because we all are so different!

If I can encourage you, we have actually had people GAIN weight on week 1 and then come back to lose a good amount by the end. So be patient with yourself and know that what you are doing is so good for your body and has long-term benefits and rewards if you do not give up!! Keep on keeping on!! This 40 Days is about so much more than numbers!!

Some people have never done a water only fast for 24 hours. If you are able, choose a day this week where you can slow your routine, spend extra time in prayer, and drink water only. Fasting will realign your appetites. The health benefits are big, but the spiritual benefits are bigger.

How are you feeling? What are you loving? What have you noticed is working better in your life over the past week? Have you thought about or viewed food differently? Write your comments and celebrate--you are progressing!!

Food Journal - *What I ate today:*

_____
_____
_____
_____
_____
_____
_____

Comments - *How did I feel today & what did I learn?*

_____
_____
_____
_____
_____
_____
_____
_____

What do I need to work on:

_____
_____
_____
_____
_____
_____
_____

Day 34

The Grief Committee

And in those days, when the number of the disciples was multiplied, there arose a murmuring of the Grecians against the Hebrews, because their widows were neglected in the daily ministration. Then the twelve called the multitude of the disciples unto them, and said, It is not reason that we should leave the word of God, and serve tables. Wherefore, brethren, look ye out among you seven men of honest report, full of the Holy Ghost and wisdom, whom we may appoint over this business. But we will give ourselves continually to prayer, and to the ministry of the word. And the saying pleased the whole multitude: and they chose Stephen, a man full of faith and of the Holy Ghost, and Philip, and Prochorus, and Nicanor, and Timon, and Parmenas, and Nicolas a proselyte of Antioch: Whom they set before the apostles: and when they had prayed, they laid their hands on them. Acts 6:1-6

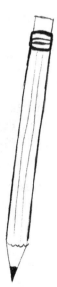

In Acts chapter 6, the newborn church, who had a multitude of needs in teaching and ministry and prayer and administration, set aside and anointed seven men, described as full of the Holy Ghost and faith and power, who did great wonders among the people. What was their job description, you ask? "See that the widows are not neglected in the daily ministry." Widows have a special place in the heart of God!

Unfortunately, I can speak about widowhood as an expert, having been widowed for the third time before the age of 50. My book, *Comfort and Joy: How to Receive Healing Beyond Grief and Loss*, is my story of how the scriptures and the church restored my life and gave me what I needed to live in victory and health. How did I do it? Well, it wasn't with chocolate and cheese cake. I cried out with David, *My heart is sore pained within me: and the terrors of death are fallen upon me. Fearfulness and trembling are come upon me, and horror hath overwhelmed me* (Psalm 55:4-5). I turned to the truth of God's word, and the comfort of the Holy Spirit, and I obeyed His commands to choose abundant life for the future He planned for me. And I found that walking in health is foundational to being a servant of the Most High God.

People often talk about modeling the modern church using the book of Acts. So I would ask you to consider if there are seven people or so in your church who are full of the Holy Ghost and faith, who would have a heart for helping those who have faced loss, or are in a health crisis and need special care now.

Grieving people need the church to help them stay out of the food trap. Whether it is death, divorce, the loss of job, or major life changes, a person can fall into a destructive pattern of not eating, or eating to medicate her depression and sorrow. Junk food and alcohol will increase her inability to cope with life. God wants our bodies to be healthy, strong and balanced, and eating is a far more spiritual decision than we admit. Could your Appetite for God group be the first accountability partners who would pray with a grieving person, walk or run with her, and encourage healthy eating and physical fitness? The grieving one needs to eat for nutrition more than ever!

One of my great needs as a widow has been to talk to another adult. After years of morning conversation about literally everything in life, there was no one over the age of twelve to talk to. I longed for someone to come to my house and sit at my table and talk to me. A widow quickly loses the "couples" friends they have had all their lives. She can't afford dinners out, and doesn't fit into their lifestyle any more. It's not that they don't care about her. But I have never talked to a single widow who maintained the same friends as she had as a married couple. Will you help her? Keeping the widow in community will protect her. Her earthly protector is gone! It is a very scary place, and probably an area of neglect. Take the example of the newborn church in Acts 8. Befriend someone who is depressed and not functioning well because of their past life circumstances or their current sugar and carb overload, and change their future of poor health and inability to work for God. God has a special place in His heart and in His church for suffering people. I am so grateful for this truth!

Health Lesson:

When you go shopping at the grocery store, you might be tempted to pick up that item that is on sale and so cheap! Remember, 70 percent of the food in the grocery store contains genetically modified ingredients—avoid that corn, soy, sugar, and canola/cottonseed oil no matter what! I know we have talked a lot about genetically modified foods, but because the research is not reported in American media as it is in other parts of the world, we have trouble understanding the scope of the problem. I am attaching one more GM food link to an article that should boost your resolve to give up that stuff forever—it is a report of peer-reviewed scientific studies that raise serious questions about the safety and ethics of GM food.

Read the article "Why Genetically Engineered Food is Dangerous: New Report by Genetic Engineers" in the multimedia section of www.AppetiteforGod.com.

WHAT TO DO:

By now your workbook should be well worn, and other recipes you have used have been added. You can make notes for substitutions and add clean healthy recipes to make this program one of a kind for you. I've found I don't use a cookbook very much since I am eating clean and simple fresh food, but recipes will help you add flavor without adding junk calories.

Do another internet search for a paleo recipe that is grain, sugar, and dairy free. You can substitute stevia for sugar, and nut flours (almond, cashew, and coconut) for grain flours. Choose a main dish to prepare this week.

Food Journal - *What I ate today:*

_____

_____

_____

_____

_____

_____

_____

_____

Comments - *How did I feel today & what did I learn?*

_____

_____

_____

_____

_____

_____

_____

_____

_____

What do I need to work on:

_____

_____

_____

_____

_____

_____

_____

_____

Day 35

How Much Strength Do You Have?

And he said unto me, My grace is sufficient for thee: for my strength is made perfect in weakness. Most gladly therefore will I rather glory in my infirmities, that the power of Christ may rest upon me. II Corinthians 12:9

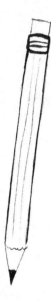

Our desire for food, and the pleasure we experience from it, begins at birth, and extends to our final days. No wonder it can hold too much power over us. No wonder we struggle to master its attraction. No wonder it has become the center of social life. Everyone's body has a fragile balance that needs particular fuel to maintain its ideal weight, metabolism, and energy. In order to reach that ideal, we must deny ourselves today's addictive sugars and altered grains that will render the body incapable of health.

Why didn't God just design us to eat one food, once a week, like we put gas in a car, or replace batteries in a flashlight? It is because food teaches us great lessons about God's grace. Humility is developed under pressure. We can use our desires for food to be thankful to God and to discipline ourselves; or we can use food to lead us to destruction. Food reminds us that we are completely dependent upon God—"when I am weak, then I am strong." When we call upon God alone to "give us daily our daily bread," we acknowledge that He is the provider of everything good, and that everything He gives us must be given back to Him in loving service. Discipline in eating is an act of love towards God. When we walk in health with strong physical bodies and clear minds, we are demonstrating that the power of God rests upon us.

John Bunyon said it most eloquently when he wrote, "The great practical question for us, in our endeavour to live the godly life, is not—What have we to bear? But—what strength have we for the bearing?

Health Lesson:

What causes high blood pressure? Here is an excerpt from *Dr. Deanna's Healing Handbook*:

Dr. Mark Houston of Vanderbilt University has written an excellent book on hypertension, which I highly recommend if you or someone you love has hypertension. He has also written a medical textbook on the topic as well. In his book, *What Your Doctor May Not Tell You About Hypertension* he helps people understand the factors that play into this disease as well as the silent damage that takes place for those who have it.

Hypertension is a manifestation of the health of the blood vessel. If a blood vessel is healthy then the blood pressure will be at or below 115/70. When the blood pressure starts to creep above that number it is an indication that there is inflammation, oxidative stress and most likely an autoimmune like state that takes place within the lining of the blood vessel.

Diseased blood vessels begin to lose elasticity and consequently blood pressure numbers begin to escalate. Think of it this way: Imagine the different rate at which water flows through a flexible garden hose versus the rate of flow through a steel pipe. If you were to apply the same amount of water pressure at the entry point of the flexible hose and the rigid metal pipe, the rigid metal pipe would have much higher pressure at the ending point and it's much the same with blood vessels. As the blood vessel becomes stiff and rigid, blood pressure numbers increase.

Treating the blood vessel starts with a diet high in protein and complex carbohydrates, all low on the glycemic index. There are many supplements that can make a dramatic difference as well. Many supplements act like natural calcium channel blockers or even ACE Inhibitors, both of which are blood pressure medications. The ones proven in studies to be of benefit are: Vitamins B6, B12, C and E, CoEnzyme Q10, Folic Acid, L-Arginine and Alpha Lipoic Acid.

WHAT TO DO:

Review the supplements you are taking. A high absorption multi-vitamin, Vitamin D-3 and Omega 3's are for everyone. If you are taking other supplements, or would like to boost your health, research the benefits of CoEnzyme Q10 and Vitamin C, or a B vitamin supplement. Our soils are depleted, and our foods are nutrient poor. It may be time for you to reconsider adding supplements to your diet.

Food Journal - *What I ate today:*

_____

_____

_____

_____

_____

_____

_____

Comments - *How did I feel today & what did I learn?*

_____

_____

_____

_____

_____

_____

_____

_____

What do I need to work on:

_____

_____

_____

_____

_____

_____

_____

Day 36

An Offering to the Lord

And the king said unto Araunah, Nay; but I will surely buy it of thee at a price: neither will I offer burnt offerings unto the LORD my God of that which doth cost me nothing. So David bought the threshing floor and the oxen for fifty shekels of silver. And David built there an altar unto the LORD, and offered burnt offerings and peace offerings. So the LORD was intreated for the land, and the plague was stayed from Israel. 2 Samuel 24:24-25

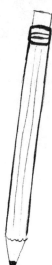

In a moment of pride, David disobeyed God by taking a census. He wanted to prove his own power, and flaunt the strength of his armies and his people. God forgave David, and told him to go to Araunah's farm and make sacrifices there to atone for his sin. Araunah was thrilled and privileged to have a visit from the king, and offered David his place, his oxen, and all that he needed to do what God asked.

David's response has stirred the heart of every Christian in the western world who lives with daily excess and a great temptation for luke-warmness and complacency. "Neither will I offer burnt offerings to the Lord my God of that which cost me nothing." True disciples of Christ will give sacrificially. There is no price too high to see God's will done on earth as it is in heaven. Those who give God only what costs them nothing have never discovered Jesus admonition, *And he said to them all, If any man will come after me, let him deny himself, and take up his cross daily, and follow me (Luke 9:23).*

There is a cost in denying our appetites to become a daily follower of Christ. He is calling us to be fit to serve. I have prayed for you as you have worked through these 40 days, that you would be a faithful and mighty laborer in God's harvest. The harvest truly is great, but the laborers are few (Luke 10:2). Do not be sidelined from the work of the Kingdom by your appetites. May you prosper and be in health, even as your soul prospers (3 John 1:2).

Health Lesson:

Alejandro Junger, M.D. wrote a book called *Clean Gut: The Breakthrough Plan for Eliminating the Root Cause of Disease and Revolutionizing Your Health.* (Harper-Collins, 2013). I am always interested in what a medical doctor has to say when the focus is the root cause of disease rather than the efficacy of a drug to treat symptoms. If you are thinking about taking a probiotic supplement, this may encourage you to get started—

The gut's good bacteria neutralize about 40 percent of the toxins we consume in our food, acting as a kind of satellite liver (p. 26). If the gut didn't have intestinal flora, the liver would have to work almost twice as hard. The gut also has a nervous system with brain-like functions. Nerve filaments send and receive messages from our gut neurons, which coordinate, modulate, and regulate gut function, including peristalsis, digestion, immunity, and hormone balance (p. 43). There are more neurotransmitters in the gut than in the brain. Serotonin, the neurotransmitter responsible for feelings of well-being are manufactured 90 percent in the gut.

Check the bibliography for books on gut health. A compendium of current gut health research is published in *Dr. Deanna's Healing Handbook.*

WHAT TO DO:

You need to track daily caloric intake throughout this 40 Days. Why? Clean, whole foods are high in nutrients, but naturally low in calories. Because of this, our bodies are satisfied, we aren't hungry and we don't even snack sometimes. In order to keep our metabolism humming, we have to be in what I call the 'sweet spot'. If you do not get adequate calories (+1200), your body will go into 'starvation mode' and you will store fat (not lose weight, maybe even gain). The body says "I don't know when s/he will feed me next, so I better hold on to this!" Anna Joy and I lost weight staying in the window between 1,000 and 1,200 calories. You should have a window by now that you stay in to keep your metabolism at its peak.

So, track your calories…just to get a good average. If you exercise, track calories on an exercise day and a non-exercise day.

FOOD calories minus EXERCISE calories = NET calories. NET calories need to be 1200+.

Ex: I ate 1200 calories and burned 400 in my exercise class. My NET is 800. Will I lose weight? Not as much as I could. If I want to keep my metabolism up and keep burning calories, and I know I'm going to burn 400 in the gym, then I need to EAT 1400 to 1600. Again, because your shakes are clean, whole foods are naturally low in calories, this may mean adding snacks, and more healthy calories like a handful of nuts between meals. Nuts, nut butters, seeds & avocados are all high in healthy fat and a quick way to pack in the calories, so use in moderation.

PS – You can use myfitnesspal.com (or the smartphone app) for tracking calories (both food & exercise).

Food Journal - *What I ate today:*

_____
_____
_____
_____
_____
_____

Comments - *How did I feel today & what did I learn?*

_____
_____
_____
_____
_____
_____
_____

What do I need to work on:

_____
_____
_____
_____
_____
_____

Day 37

Glorify God With Your Body

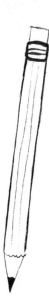

What? know ye not that your body is the temple of the Holy Ghost which is in you, which ye have of God, and ye are not your own? For ye are bought with a price: therefore glorify God in your body, and in your spirit, which are God's. I Corinthians 6:19-20

The stories of Belshazzar in the Old Testament, and Herod in the New Testament are sobering condemnations, as their sin was identified thus: "They gave not God the glory." God commands us to use our bodies to glorify Him. To glorify God in my body means to provide for my own health to the extent that my body will function to accomplish God's perfect will. It is not an obsession with beauty or body building. It is not focusing on the body merely for the body's sake. After all, our bodies belong to God alone.

You know that a sugar-free GMO-free diet will improve your health. You know that 20 minutes of moderate exercise every day will give you stronger stamina and thought. What are you waiting for? Each time you are tempted to put toxins in your body, remember you are handing poison to God's property. You bring glory to Him when you care for your health, taking action on what you know to be true. Food is fuel. To God be the glory!

Health Lesson:

One of the most important keys to sustainable weight loss, health and energy is keeping your blood sugar stable. When you eat low glycemic index foods, your blood sugar never gets too high or too low. This keeps your metabolism stable and tames those unhealthy cravings for sweets and salt. Of course, when it comes to blood sugar and a healthy weight, what you eat is just as important as how often you eat. Skip the "high glycemic" foods that cause your blood sugar to spike, like bread, sugar, fruit juices and processed carbohydrates.

You feel like you haven't eaten at all only an hour or two later? Then, choose lots of lean proteins, healthy fats, and "low glycemic" fruits and vegetables. Add quinoa once or twice a week if you are craving carbs. If your insulin levels are unstable, as evidenced by needing a nap every time you eat, feeling foggy or shaky before a meal, or dizziness following a sugar/bread snack, you may need to alter your diet to a very low level of carbs to break the cycles of leptin and insulin resistance. Dr. Ron Rosedale has been writing about this issue for decades, and his book, *The Rosedale Diet*, is helpful in coaching diabetics and heart patients to better nutrition.

WHAT TO DO:

Mix up a batch of protein bars from your protein powder, and keep a few in your car in a zip lock. Be prepared to have a protein snack when you get hungry. If stabilizing your blood sugar is a concern, add a tsp. of cinnamon to your shakes each morning to lower your blood sugar naturally.

Food Journal - *What I ate today:*

_____
_____
_____
_____
_____
_____
_____

Comments - *How did I feel today & what did I learn?*

_____
_____
_____
_____
_____
_____
_____
_____

What do I need to work on:

_____
_____
_____
_____
_____
_____
_____

Day 38

Desiring Bread

Neither let us tempt Christ, as some of them also tempted, and were destroyed of serpents. Neither murmur ye, as some of them also murmured, and were destroyed of the destroyer. I Corinthians 10:9-10

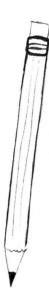

I know the story of the Exodus well, and I Corinthians 10 is all about how the Israelites gave us an example so we wouldn't mess up like they did. God gave miracles to them in deliverance, in food, in clothing that didn't wear out, in winning battles, and in healing. Then Paul says they tempted Christ and were destroyed by snakebite. I'm sure glad they haven't made a Christian movie about that—nightmares! Once I get past the picture in my mind of poisonous snakes appearing in a crowd, I think, "But wait a minute! That was 4,000 years before Christ." At first glance it looks like the beatings and imprisonments are getting to Paul's chronological memory. He says they tempted Christ! The amplified explanation is this: "They tried His patience, became a trial to Him, critically appraised Him, and exploited His goodness." Right along with their sins of idolatry and immorality, Paul puts his finger on their murmuring and complaining about their food as sins against Christ. They devalued His gifts to them, and scorned His love for them with their whining for something different.

I needed to dig deeper. What about the "fiery serpents" that bit the people? It's a brief reference from Numbers 21:5-6. The words they spoke that displeased Christ were this: "our soul loathes this worthless bread." Manna had no flavor enhancers or processed sugar to excite the taste buds or the brain. It was body fuel. Period. And they had no gratitude for the manna that appeared every morning that sustained them in their journey.

Suddenly I understood Paul's reference to tempting Christ. The manna was their bread of life. And Paul, knowing Jesus' final hours when He broke bread, and said "this is my body," and comprehending Jesus' title as the "Bread of Life," he writes that the sin of the Israelites that warranted death by snakebite was this—they despised the bread that gave them life.

I might have missed it thinking I'd never be walking in a desert for 40 years, so the admonition didn't apply to me. But Paul brought Jesus into the warning, and suddenly, the word is as fresh as the sunrise. My flesh cries out for more than food as fuel. Who hasn't started their morning with a dozen hot donuts, or ended their dinner with triple-chocolate dark devil's food cake? I complain about the "worthless bread," that builds my body at the cellular level, and is a miraculous gift from the Savior's hand. I live an empty spiritual appetite that denies the Bread of Life that feeds my soul and spirit, and gives me all things I need.

I held my breath as I read Numbers 11—a whole chapter about the whining and complaining. Moses got so sick of their carping, he went to the Lord and said, "I didn't give birth to this bunch of babies. Just let me die!" And God lifted his burden and gave the people more, in spite of their ungrateful hearts.

"The Lord will give you flesh, and ye shall eat. Ye shall not eat one day, nor two days, nor five days, neither ten days, nor twenty days; But even a whole month, until it come out at your nostrils, and it be loathsome unto you: because that ye have despised the Lord which is among you, and have wept before him, saying, Why came we forth out of Egypt?" That picture is about as gross as the slithering snakes.

Lord, please don't send in the snakes. Forgive my wandering heart. I loathe my sin that questions Your care for me. I have tried Your patience with my senseless scurrying for more. I have exploited Your goodness by careless eating and being content with provision for only myself, while the world around me trembles with hunger for the Bread of Life. Thank you for visiting me in the quietness of the morning, for sending your Holy Spirit to redirect my heart to love You, and to shake away the unstable double-mindedness that denies Your care for me. Today I entrust myself to Your keeping, and I celebrate that I am fed my ordinary bread and the Bread of Life. I am privileged to know the love of Christ, which is beyond knowledge, and I am filled with all the fullness of God (Ephesians 3:19). My appetite is for You, God!

Health Lesson:

In 2012, a pediatric pulmonologist at Akron Children's Hospital published an article in the scientific journal, *Pediatrics*, stating that acetaminophen, or Tylenol, is contributing to the rise in asthma cases. "If people say they take acetaminophen once a month, generally their risk of having asthma has doubled." The rate of asthma more than doubled from 1980 to 1994, and by 2009, the government reported that 8.2 percent of Americans have asthma. An August, 2010 New York Times article reported that teens who use acetaminophen once a month develop asthma symptoms more than twice as often as those who don't take it. The data represented 322,000 children ages 13 and 14 from 50 countries.

Every drug we take, whether over the counter or prescription, changes our bodies at the cellular level. We should limit our intake of pharmaceuticals for minor discomfort, and allow the body's immune system to do what God designed it to do. Dr. Natasha Campbell-McBride reminds parents that chicken soup and cold liquids can provide the needed comfort that gives the body time to heal itself.

WHAT TO DO:

If you take antihistamines during allergy season, choose one that is free of the unneeded addition of acetaminophen. Know the side effects of every pharmaceutical you use. As Hippocrates advised us 400 years before Christ, "Let food be thy medicine and medicine thy food." If you know someone who is  frustrated with weight gain, or has given up hope of improving their health, why not invite them to consider their Appetite for God? When Anna Joy and I transformed our bodies and our lives, other family members joined in, and people naturally asked "What happened to you!!!" We love it when people tell us they've heard our story!

Go to the multimedia section of the www.AppetiteforGod.com and watch the video, My Story.

Food Journal - *What I ate today:*

_____
_____
_____
_____
_____
_____
_____

Comments - *How did I feel today & what did I learn?*

_____
_____
_____
_____
_____
_____
_____
_____

What do I need to work on:

_____
_____
_____
_____
_____
_____
_____

Day 39

The Mindset of Health

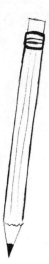

Wherefore gird up the loins of your mind, be sober, and hope to the end for the grace that is to be brought unto you at the revelation of Jesus Christ. I Peter 1:13

God has work He planned for us before we were born (Ephesians 2:10), but there is preparation that must be done in order to complete His plan for our lives. Planning requires clear thinking, anticipating the action required, and gathering the necessary materials, choosing the location, and setting into motion the action that will be accomplished. Most of us set out with schemes that take unexpected turns. That's where the grace of God comes in. We can place our hopes fully and completely on God to help us with clear thinking, healthy brains, good logic, and adequate foresight to accomplish His will. But consider—we have a responsibility in the process.

This verse starts with what WE do. Feed your brain the fuel it needs to live! Let's prepare our minds to be healthy and functioning to the glory of God for every day we live on this earth!

Health Lesson:

According to the National Institutes of Health, one fourth of American's suffer from depression, and over twelve billion dollars are spent for antidepressants annually. The more we understand about the gut-brain connection, the clearer it is that nutrition plays a major role in depression. A meta-analysis of studies in 2010 showed a strong correlation between depression and obesity, both of which have a root of systemic inflammation. Our fat tissues release inflammatory cytokines which play a role in insulin resistance and cardiovascular disease. They can also cause inflammation in the brain. Insulin resistance causes a cascading effect—Insulin resistance causes sympathetic nervous system over stimulation, which increases cortisol levels, which causes the body to lose magnesium. This can lead to migraine headaches and insomnia.

 The intake of refined sugar has a similar effect, causing excess glucose, which degenerates brain function and causes an overproduction of cortisol. Increased cortisol has been linked to weight gain. There has been an increase in sugar intake from 2 pounds a year in 1940 to 150 pounds a year in many of today's teens who drink daily soft drinks.

Systemic inflammation can also be caused by food intolerance, especially wheat gluten, dairy and nuts. People with celiac disease report higher levels of depression. Lactose [dairy] intolerance has been linked to malabsorption of tryptophan. This leads to a serotonin deficiency, clinical depression, anxiety, and ADD/ADHD. A similar reaction can be caused by high fructose corn syrup.

Vitamin deficiency including Vitamin D and selenium contribute to depression. Addressing the root cause of depression should be done in three steps:

1. Restore adequate Vitamin D levels

2. Balance hormones, especially cortisol; remove stress and use a bioidentical hormone cream

3. Restore gut health, eliminating genetically modified foods that damage gut flora and reduce tryptophan levels, which is the precursor of serotonin. Ninety-five percent of serotonin is produced by gut flora metabolism, and is responsible for our sense of well being.

WHAT TO DO:

The tiny blood vessels in our brains can become compromised, and we don't know it until the damage is advanced. We need to raise our heart rates and MOVE for 20 minutes every day. Make a commitment to walk a mile, and get a few days head start. If your weather doesn't permit, you can find a free indoor track at a church or walk in a nearby mall. I know treadmills are not as good as walking in fresh air, but I love my treadmill for the convenience. Find a way to get that heart rate up. Buy a low impact exercise video and join in! Choose your method today for getting in that all important exercise.

TIME TO WEIGH IN! You made it! Today is the last day to record your weight and measurements. Use the chart on page 154.

Food Journal - *What I ate today:*

_____
_____
_____
_____
_____
_____
_____

Comments - *How did I feel today & what did I learn?*

_____
_____
_____
_____
_____
_____
_____
_____

What do I need to work on:

_____
_____
_____
_____
_____
_____
_____

Day 40

Final Thoughts on Gluttony

And put a knife to thy throat, if thou be a man given to appetite... Be not among winebibbers; among riotous eaters of flesh: For the drunkard and the glutton shall come to poverty: and drowsiness shall clothe a man with rags. Proverbs 23:2, 20-21

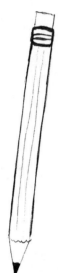

Proverbs 23 is a litany of warnings about our human appetites. In this chapter Solomon declares it is better to have a knife at your throat than to be captive to uncontrolled eating.

Reaching back to the 1800's, Dr. E. Johnson writes, "gluttony has been pointed to as the source of our infirmities, the fountain of all our diseases. As a lamp is choked by superabundance of oil, a fire extinguished by excess of fuel, so is the natural heat of the body destroyed by intemperate diet. By slow degrees, and more and more, the habits of self-indulgence undermine the strength of body, still more certainly the vigor of mind, until poverty comes like an armed man."

And now in the 21st century, scholars from major research universities the world over are affirming that a diet that spikes the blood sugar does indeed undermine our strength and vigor of mind. Drowsiness that we are warned about in this proverb often occurs after eating, and is a clear signal of unhealthy fluctuation of blood sugar. Processed sugar, grains, high glycemic index foods, and simple carbohydrates chronically overload the body, eventually leading to insulin resistance and diabetes.

When the blood sugar remains high more than two hours after a meal, the risk for dementia is doubled. If your overeating is producing drowsiness, your body is signaling DANGER. You must choose foods that fuel your body in health rather than assault your body with sugar overload.

The final warning is that drowsiness will end in poverty. God wants you to be productive, energetic, and working full of vigor to build His kingdom. It requires a healthy body. Through fasting and prayer and choosing body fuel foods, we can put a knife to the uncontrolled appetites that are robbing us of our goal—"Fit to Serve with an Appetite for God!"

Health Lesson:

To understand more fully the damage done by sugar and simple carbs, here is an excerpt from *Dr. Deanna's Healing Handbook*:

Insulin Resistance

If you lack energy, wonder often if you're "coming down with something," and fight fatigue every day, you may be struggling with insulin resistance. Insulin resistance occurs when cells fail to respond to the hormone insulin. This happens when the body has been forced to produce a large amount of insulin in response to continuous, on-going high glycemic load, which is caused by eating too much sugar and refined carbs and the system eventually wears down and then out! Insulin resistance (IR) rides along for years wearing down energy and productivity levels. IR has increased dramatically in the past 10 years rising along with the rates of metabolic syndrome in the US.

Metabolic syndrome can be signaled by fogginess and inability to focus; high blood sugar; intestinal bloating – as most intestinal gas is produced from carbohydrates that humans do not digest and absorb well; sleepiness, especially after meals; weight gain, fat storage, difficulty losing weight – for most people, excess weight is from high fat storage; the fat of Insulin Resistance is generally stored in and around abdominal organs in both males and females and it is likely that hormones produced in that fat are a precipitating cause of insulin resistance, increased blood triglyceride levels, and increased blood pressure. Three out of four Americans today are either overweight or obese and a staggering thirty percent of US children are also overweight or obese.

According to an article in *The New England Journal of Medicine*, it is estimated 91 percent of diabetes could be prevented if people followed a low glycemic diet (low carbs and sugars) and got 30 minutes of vigorous exercise daily.(N Eng J Med 2001;(11):790-797). Again, the solution is literally at the end of our forks in most cases!

WHAT TO DO:

Mix up a fresh batch of protein bars and pick up some Granny Smith apples and organic berries. You can snack a bit and still keep your system clean. I like vanilla protein bars for variety. The recipe is below.

- 4 cups Vanilla Pea Protein
- 1 15 oz. can coconut milk
- 2 TB almond butter
- 1 tsp. almond extract

Mix and press into 9 X 13 pan and sprinkle generously with cinnamon. Cut into 20 bars, each about 75 calories.

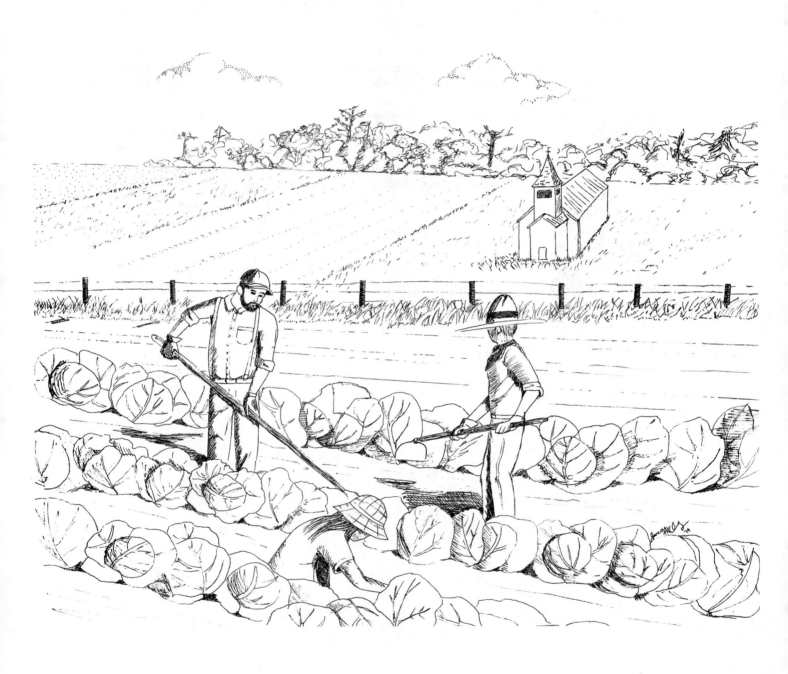

Concluding remarks

Returning to the Garden

During this 40 Day adventure we have sought to reestablish an Appetite for God and an appetite for food that brings glory to God and makes us fit for service. It is our hope and prayer that you are now thinking about your ordinary and necessary food in a new way. The distance between the garden and the table should be much shorter. We have a great appreciation for God's careful planning for clean water, rich soil, and life giving sun, and His gift of the seed which is fruitful and nourishing from generation to generation.

Though now the church takes the lead in obesity and chronic disease, we have a great opportunity to give witness to God's gift of health in a world that is becoming sicker every day. As I drive through the countryside and see old stone churches with tall tomb stones covering the yard, I am reminded that the church has always cared for people in death. I long to see the day when driving in the countryside, every church has cultivated its unused land and is teeming with fruits and vegetables that are clean, free of pesticides and herbicides, and non-GMO. Who can give life and health to our children? As my three-year-old grandson watches the seeds he planted producing a hundred-fold, we talk about faith as the grain of a mustard seed, the patience of God like the farmer waiting for rain, and the importance of abiding in the vine in order to have life.

Here is the promise of Jesus in his final hours with his disciples,

> *Abide in me, and I in you. As the branch cannot bear fruit of itself, except it abide in the vine, no more can ye, except ye abide in me. I am the vine, ye are the branches; He that abideth in me, and I in him, the same bringeth forth much fruit: for without me ye can do nothing. John 15:4-5*

The sad and lifeless fruit can be seen in the "nominal Christian" who does not abide in Christ, as well as in the sad and lifeless fruit of the soil, depleted of nutrition and genetically altered to be foreign to the body and to yield death to the next generation.

Why did God explain in the very beginning about seeds, and the life they contain? As man worked the land, God kept him mindful of his dependence upon the Lord of creation. He would draw nourishment from the world over which he had dominion. R. A. Redford, a 19th century pastor wrote, "If there be in man's world a contradiction between the multiplication of life and the happiness of life, it is a sign of departure from the original order." Our food was given to us by the hand of God in Genesis 1. The gardener takes joy in his work, saving the seed in which God placed life, and carrying God's order from generation to generation. God is a Master Gardener. Let's partner with Him to receive our Daily Bread.

Where Do We Go From Here

After talking with hundreds of people for whom weight loss has been a lifelong failing endeavor – like my own daughter who always ended up gaining more weight even after a successful few months of weight loss--I want to tell you what makes this plan permanent. For me, it was understanding how important health is to God.

Gardening that yielded a daily provision of food was His idea, and for me there was an unexpected deep spiritual satisfaction in joining His plan for health. However, in the joining it became clear to us that a full year was needed to overcome the unique obstacles every struggling overweight person faces: The winter blahs, holiday dinners, birthday celebrations, embarrassment at summer parties, sweet treats of ice cream and cookies for evenings alone, church potlucks, and all-you-can-eat restaurant buffets—at each season of the year traditions that bar our success must be addressed with prayer, wisdom and resolve.

Like Jesus, our appetite for God must always supersede our appetite for food (John 4:34). I will seek first the Kingdom of God, realizing it is not meat and drink, but rather righteousness, peace and joy in the Holy Spirit (Romans 14:17). The peace and joy come from knowing that the pleasures I gave up to get healthy were also the things that kept me from fully experiencing God's kingdom in my life.

Today I face each new challenge by thanking God for my provision of "necessary and ordinary" daily food that has broken my cravings and appetites that eventually lead to chronic disease and early death. With knowledge and understanding, today I am resolved to walk through each season of the year surrendering my appetites to God, while giving an example of victorious living and thereby helping others to become fit for life and service. Start every day this year thanking God for what you have learned and can put into practice. Your gratitude will satisfy you and keep your appetites in line!

Today, I encourage you to detox by enjoying your two shakes and one meal as you already have for these 40 days, gathering strength to make good confessions and prevail during the months ahead and all seasonal challenges. With God's help, it is up to you. "I can do all things through Christ Who strengthens me!"

If you have reached your ideal weight, you may want to switch to one shake a day, and two clean meals. Or, if you want to take off an additional ten or fifteen more pounds, you can decide to keep going with the detoxing protein supplement program. Anna Joy and I used the two shakes and 1 meal regimen for about four months; then I switched to one shake a day and two meals. When I am busy, I still fix two shakes a day if I don't have time to eat clean food – it's my new "fast food."

Most of us who have participated in the *Appetite for God* program are part of a family. Our decisions don't affect just ourselves, and for a few, if it was only about them, they don't care enough about themselves to do what is necessary to become healthy. If you have doubts, I would like for you to carefully consider the final section of *An Appetite for God*, which is a compendium of research on childhood diseases that have skyrocketed in the last decade. If we wouldn't change our eating habits for ourselves, we must make these changes for our children, who are the first generation in history predicted to live shorter lives than their parents. If this were a plague like the cholera and black plagues of other centuries, we would not hesitate to protect ourselves from the assault. Our vulnerable children need that kind of protection and provision from parents for their future health and well being. You cannot deprive your children of junk food; you can only save them from it. The success of *An Appetite for God* will be measured by a generation that has escaped crushing, debilitating disease and walks in health, from the youngest to the oldest. Consider this information on children's health, and if you have a loved one who is suffering from asthma, ADHD, or autism, I would urge you to consult the bibliography for further resources.

Our transformation and return to the garden and ordinary and necessary food is so full of wonder and joy. I cannot express how grateful to God I am when I hear Anna Joy say, "it's a 30 YEAR program!" We have left chronic disease and early death behind and will keep reaching higher and higher for a cleaner, nutrient richer, healthful lifestyle. You will not be sorry this part of your life is redeemed. I'm so glad you joined us!

Children's Health

Protecting Our Children
Allergies, Asthma, ADHD, Autism

I talk to many people who are finally examining their health needs because a family member is in crisis. Mom has cancer. Little Josh has asthma. Mary has acne. Dad is struggling to work because of high blood pressure and migraine headaches. I got healthy because of a teenager daughter in crisis. She was seventeen and moving rapidly towards 300 pounds. The prom dress shopping disaster and the questions about stomach stapling jolted me to find a permanent solution to the problem that was destroying my daughter, physically, emotionally and spiritually. Two years later when I look in the mirror, I realize the one who benefited the most was me. That's because I'm the grocery shopper and the cook; I can teach my children and grandchildren to live in health and never face the chronic illnesses that are diet driven.

If you are doing this program for yourself, please don't be a short order cook and serve up junk to your family. Ask them to get healthy for you, just for 40 days, and then you all can get healthy together. Yes, you will deal with resistance. My oldest child was 29 and my youngest 15 when I started this program. They were the two who resisted the hardest. My youngest, who is now 17, is a gourmet grain free cook, and she is FINALLY working on her own health. It was a long road. I love it when my grandsons fight over broccoli and swiss chard smoothies. They have never tasted fast food junk. My biggest problem is keeping Caleb, now three, from pulling up a bean plant in the garden when I've turned my head. Do this for the children. There are no regrets!

Many people awaken to their need for better health around fifty years of age, when the results of toxic overload begin to manifest themselves in the form of a chronic life-shortening disease. Then drastic measures are required to regain an acceptable level of functional health, because years of inflammation, carbohydrate overload, and toxin ingestion have measurably and negatively impacted the function of the brain, gut and major organs. But the health problems are not a sudden body shift. We develop and pass on to our children abnormal health from the moment they are born.

When a baby is born, the gut is sterile, and the infant is dependent on his mother to populate the gut with healthy bacteria. Mothers in their childbearing years can pass along to their babies an abnormal and poorly functioning immunity, which is the result of years of assault on the normal gut flora from environmental factors, personal care products, genetically modified food and toxic food additives. The baby starts life with a below-the-baseline immunity inherited from Mom. Antibiotics are frequently given in the first year of life which further diminishes the function of the gut flora, which are responsible for 80 percent of our immunity. It is little wonder with 40+/- vaccines introduced in infancy, children are unable to recover from such an overload, and in record numbers today manifest the "4 As" – allergies, asthma, ADHD and Autism.

Given the routine challenges today, our children will only be healthy if we address their cellular needs beginning before conception and then into adulthood. This 40-Day Fitness Program is a family affair—not just for the 50-somethings who are battling inflammation, fatigue, hormone imbalance, and premature aging. How can we help our children avoid the epidemic of childhood diseases that have suddenly skyrocketed in their generation?

Children require the same basic nutritional fuel as adults. Metabolic balance, detoxification, clean food and a toxin-free environment protect all of us from chronic illness caused by toxic overload on the body. If we begin now, and protect our children even in the womb, we can avoid some of the heart ache we see in suffering children all around us. When skin disorders, learning disabilities, and obesity are visible, we know there are invisible problems at the cellular level that can be addressed. The earlier we take action, the sooner our children will experience freedom from disease, and the health and energy all children should possess.

How the Body Stays Healthy

The body's autoimmune response is a careful balance of T-cell function, which are white blood cells produced by the thymus. Some of these cells kill cancer cells, some stimulate the immune response, and some turn it off after the health crisis is solved. Two helper T-cells, Th-1 and Th-2, are important for a strong immune system. Th-1 cells attack pathogens directly that are lodged inside infected cells. Th-2 cells send messages that enhance the immune system's ability to produce antibodies. Th-2 cells do not enter an infected cell, but when the two immune helpers are balanced and in sync, the body's ability to fight disease is optimized.

Yeast overgrowth, and the presence of mercury, aluminum and other heavy metals skew the immune response towards Th-2 cells. The immune system becomes overexcited, resulting in allergies and autoimmune disease where the body attacks healthy tissues and organs. In Th-2 dominance, the body struggles to fight off viruses, bacteria and fungal infection. The result is widespread inflammation that may present itself as respiratory or skin allergies, asthma, and food allergies. Kids with ADHD and autism tend to be Th-2 skewed, and in asthma, the Th-2 skewing is most extreme.[1]

The following disorders have an allergic component: ADHD, arthritis, asthma, candidiasis, chronic ear infections, chronic fatigue syndrome, depression, anxiety, hyperactivity, diabetes, digestive upset, food cravings, eczema, acne, hives, fibromyalgia, hay fever, headaches, hypoglycemia, insomnia, IBS, obesity, and sinusitis. The three main sources of asthmatic inflammation are infection such as chronic yeast, or lingering viral or bacterial infection; allergens, the most common of which are milk and wheat; and toxins, most commonly heavy metals found in vaccines and outdoor pollution.

Incidence

Kaiser Health Care, who treated 842,830 kids during the research period, reported in the *Journal of the American Medical Association Pediatrics* that ADHD has risen 24% from 2001 to 2010, and in the March 2012 issue of *Academic Pediatrics*, researchers from Northwestern Medicine reported a 66% increase in ADHD in 10 years. Researchers report these affected children have 50% less tryptophan in the gut than non-ADHD children. Normal tryptophan levels depend on our gut flora's ability to metabolize proteins. As of April, 2012 reported in *The New York Times*, ADHD affects 1 in 5 high school boys, and 6.4 million children have received the ADHD diagnosis, which is a 53 percent increase in ten years. Two-thirds of them are taking stimulants such as Ritalin and Alderol.

A 2013 study from the Kennedy Krieger Institute showed that a third of children with autism spectrum disorders also showed clinically significant symptoms of ADHD. On March 13, 2013, the CDC announced a 72 percent increase in the diagnosis of autism over the past four years. On March 27, 2014 the CDC announced a 30 percent increase in autism from 2012, from 1 in 88 children to 1 in 66 children in 2014. The incidence is almost five times as high in boys, now 1 in 44 boys. I cannot imagine a more alarming statistic, which was reported by the media with a yawn. Based on worldwide peer reviewed large scale research studies, we know several risk factors that are damaging our children's gut bacteria, resulting in a completely inadequate immune system. Because the richest and most powerful companies in the world will not act on their behalf, we as parents, grandparents and members of the body of Christ are responsible to save our children from the suffering all around us.

Finally, childhood cancer is also rising. One in every 330 American children gets cancer. From the early 80's to the early 90's, cancer in children under 10 rose 37 percent. The National Cancer Institute reported that, for infants less than one year old, the cancer rate increased 36 percent during the years 1976-84 to the years 1986-94. The greatest percentage increase occurred for germ cell cancers (increase of 124%), central nervous system cancers (increase of 57%), liver cancers (increase of 50%), and neuroblastoma (increase of 35%).

---

1   Kenneth Bock, M.D., *Healing the New Childhood Epidemics*. Ballantine Books, 2007, pp. 127-161.

Risk Factors

Children inheriting compromised and weakened gut flora from their mothers find these further assaults to their immune system significantly challenging. Given the compromised guts of most infants today, the multiple exposures to processed and GMO food, massive intake of refined GMO sugar, false estrogens and toxins in personal care products, and the number of vaccines and the heavy metals they contain overwhelm their immune systems. The following risk factors have been confirmed in worldwide research studies, and give parents guidance in protecting their children and restoring families to health.

1. Candida overgrowth

Candida in small amounts in the intestine is normal, but must be kept in check by beneficial yeast and bacteria. Antibiotics, chlorine, and birth control pills destroy friendly bacteria while leaving the Candida intact. Sugar and refined carbs encourage its growth, which is especially a problem for children.

According to Dr. Mark Hyman, the average kid in America consumes about 34 teaspoons of sugar daily. The overgrowth becomes worse during pregnancy because Candida thrives on progesterone which is at a much higher level during pregnancy.

Candida overgrowth is transferred from mother to baby during birth. It changes to a fungal form which drills holes in the intestinal wall and causes a condition known as "leaky gut." This activates the immune system to attack particles of undigested food that get through the wall of the small intestine and into the bloodstream resulting in food allergies.

Fungal overgrowth also prevents the proper digestion of protein, including the most important protein, glutathione, the body's main cellular detoxifier. The liver uses it to clean the blood and the lungs use it to clean the air. Glutathione also acts as a virus killer. The body and brain are not detoxified when glutathione is lacking.[2] Yeast in the amniotic fluid paralyzes the gut wall, and results in infant constipation.

2. Vaccines and exposure to heavy metals[3]

In male infants vaccinated at birth with thimerosal-containing HBV, the risk of immediate developmental delays, the need for early intervention services and autism is increased anywhere from three to eight fold.[4]

Seventeen of the current 36 vaccines given to children contain aluminum, which impairs the body's ability to excrete mercury and impairs glutathione synthesis. Aluminum toxicity is also linked to symptoms associated with Parkinson's, ALS, and Alzheimer's.

Several clinical studies support the link between vaccines and asthma. A UK study reported 10.7 percent of children receiving a Pertussis vaccine developed asthma, compared to 2 percent who didn't receive the vaccine. This is true of the DTaP which replaced the DPT a few years ago. The new vaccine has only parts of the Pertussis bacteria in an effort to lessen the fever reaction that occurred with the DPT containing the whole bacteria. The new vaccine is still plagued with adverse reactions. In a US study, children vaccinated with DTaP were twice as likely to develop asthma as those who weren't.

2   http://www.ncbi.nlm.nih.gov/pmc/articles/PMC2809421/

3   J.B. Adams, et al. Mercury, lead, and zinc in baby teeth of children with autism vs. controls. *Journal of Toxicology and Environmental Health.* June 2007, 70(12): 1046-51.

4   http://www.ageofautism.com/2009/09/blockbuster-primate-study-shows-significant-harm-from-one-birth-dose-of-a-mercurycontaining-vaccine.html

Vaccinations may have caused not only systemic inflammation from heavy metals, but also may have contributed to immune skewing, and to the creation of low-level chronic infections.[5]

On March 27, 2014 the CDC announced that there has been a 30 percent increase in autism since 2012, with autism now affecting 1 in 44 boys. Autism's cause is complex, and rooted in allergies, asthma, and ADHD. One clear predisposing factor is antibiotics in the first year of life. When a baby is given antibiotics, it damages the gut flora's ability to metabolize proteins into amino acids that can be utilized by the cells for metabolism. Antibiotics decrease the baby's ability to excrete heavy metals. With twenty-six vaccines scheduled in the first fifteen months of life, the heavy metals have a cumulative effect. Vaccines now contain aluminum to "enhance" the immune response, which skews the balance of white blood cells and aluminum increases the effect of mercury toxicity. Mercury is still present in flu shots, which are recommended for pregnant women. The following chart documents that a child following the CDC recommended vaccine schedule would receive a full teaspoon of aluminum by injection, a substance which has been banned from cookware for its toxicity!

Aluminum Content of Infant Vaccines

Vaccine	When given	Aluminum per dose
Hepatitis B	Birth, 2 mo., 6 mo.	250 mcg.
DTaP	2, 4, 5, and 15 mo.	625 mcg.
Hib	2, 4, and 12 mo.	225 mcg.
Pneumococcal PCV	2, 4, 6, and 12 mo.	125 mcg.
Hep A	12, 18 mo.	250 mcg.

Dr. Natasha Campbell McBride has studied and written extensively on childhood ADHD, autism, schizophrenia, and depression. She states that the epidemic of childhood diseases have one thing in common—a compromised immune system, which cannot react to environmental threats the way children responded a generation ago. She cites to vaccines and the enormous strain they place on an already compromised immune system. McBride has found that symptoms of autism appear equally after the diphtheria-pertussis-tetanas (DPT) and the measles-mumps-rubella (MMR) vaccines. Mumps, whether exposed to the vaccine or the disease, also causes blood pressure to rise, and increased blood pressure opens the blood brain barrier allowing the virus to reach the brain. Severe headaches are a side effect of the mumps vaccine.

Vaccines may not represent a single cause, but rather "the last straw" which deepens damage already done to the immune system, and causes symptoms to appear. McBride proposes that the "vaccinate every child" rule must be changed and only after a comprehensive health history is obtained on the baby and a urine and stool analysis done to determine the risk of gut dysbiosis and the baby's immune status. Here are her recommendations:

- Vaccines may be given to healthy infants with healthy parents and whose tests show normal immune development, given in single vaccines only. A child doesn't get three childhood diseases at once in the environment. The immune system should not be overloaded artificially with multiple vaccines at once.

- Delay vaccines when the mother is healthy, but baby shows abnormalities in the immune system. They could be retested every six to eight months and vaccinated with single vaccines only when they are ready, and at least six weeks apart.

---

5   Kenneth Bock, M.D., *Healing the New Childhood Epidemics*. Ballantine Books, 2007, p. 144.

- No vaccines should be given to an infant born to a mother with allergic, autoimmune, neurological, or digestive problems. An infant with eczema, asthma, digestive problems or any disorder suggesting a compromised immune system cannot recover from vaccines. Avoid also in younger siblings of children with asthma, allergies, ADHD, epilepsy, and insulin dependent diabetes.

3. Lyme disease

The *Borrelia* bacteria that causes lyme disease can be transmitted from mother to child. *Borrelia* goes to the brain and produces toxins, which cannot be removed in a glutathione deficient autistic child.

4. Biofilms

Biofilms are a web built by bacteria which then shed their outer membrane making them unidentifiable to the immune system. Heavy metals as well as calcium magnesium and iron are used by bacteria to build biofilms. When the gut flora are out of balance, biofilms can be constructed by overgrowth opportunistic bacteria and yeast such as *E. coli*, *Streptococcus*, and *Candida*. Treatment with papaya enzyme, and a heavy metal chelator have shown promise in overcoming their resistance.

5. Viral infection during and after pregnancy[6]

Chronic viral infections affect the myelin sheath surrounding the nerves in the brain, and further damage occurs from the autoimmune response that follows. Early signs of brain damage indicate the sensory system is overloaded and in pain, which causes head beating, spinning, and repetitive motions.

6. Genetics

There is a genetic predisposition to the inability to make glutathione, which makes the autistic individual unable to detoxify. Glutathione is present in every cell in the body, and is the body's main cellular detoxifier. The genetic trigger is pulled by *Candida* overgrowth or other abnormal gut maladies, which combine with the genetic predisposition to damage the brain. A study reported in the British Medical Journal, *Lancet*, stated that ADHD, autism, and schizophrenia, depression, and bipolar disorder have the same genetic markers indicating a deficit in calcium channel activity.[7]

7. Early exposure to antibiotics

The Journal of Toxicology and Environmental Health, June 2007, states "antibiotic use is known to almost completely inhibit mercury excretion in rats due to alteration of gut flora. Thus, higher use of oral antibiotics in the children with autism may have reduced their ability to excrete mercury… and may also partially explain the high incidence of chronic gastrointestinal problems in individuals with autism."

Babies are often given antibiotics for ear infection, which does not solve the problem of abnormal bacterial flora in the mouth and eustachian tubes, and will often make the problem worse by further damaging an already abnormal flora. Dr. McBride recommends the removal of dairy, sugars, and processed carbohydrates from the diet, which feed the pathogenic flora. Then at night after brushing the teeth, open a capsule of probiotics and put the powder on the tongue. The probiotic bacteria will work on the flora of the mouth and throat all night, as well as in the back of the nose and mouth, repopulating the tonsil area with good flora. As tonsils return to normal size and open

6   California Institute of Technology. (2013, Dec. 10). "Autism-like behaviors in mice alleviated by probiotic therapy. http://www. medicalnewstoda.com/releases/269828.
7   Fitzgerald, Kelly. "Five major psychiatric disorders share genetic link." Feb. 2013, www.medicalnewstoday.com/articles/257039.

the eustachian tubes, mucus can drain from the middle ear and the constant chain of ear infections will stop.[8] This author discovered experientially that the same procedure works for adults!

8. Low Vitamin D

Vitamin D_3 is necessary for normal brain development, especially during fetal development. Pregnant women and infants need adequate exposure to the sun. African Americans do not absorb as much Vitamin D producing sunlight. Vitamin D increases glutathione levels. The primary route for brain toxicity is glutathione depletion.

9. Autoimmune Response[9]

Chronic viral and bacterial infection can wear out the immune system resulting in inflammation which further damages the myelin sheath in nerve cells, as well as the lining of the digestive tract. Associations with autism were confirmed in 2009 regarding a family history of type 1 diabetes and a maternal history of rheumatoid arthritis and celiac disease.

10. Food allergies

When the body's T-cells are overactive, the result is allergies. When an individual is unable to break down casein, the milk protein found in all dairy products, it can be absorbed by areas of the brain leading to dysfunction. Children with the "four A disorders" have a digestive disorder, and are unable to process the onslaught of sugar and carbohydrates that make up the major portion of our food in the Western world.

Dr. Sidney Valentine Haas, born in 1870, developed the diet which helped thousands of patients with multiple digestive disorders, including celiac and Crohn's disease. The same basic diet he proposed is necessary to correct the gut dysbiosis epidemic today. He and his colleagues found that patients with digestive problems could tolerate protein and fat, but complex carbohydrates from grains and starchy vegetables made the problems worse. Sugar, lactose, and other complex sugars had to be excluded. His book, *The Management of Celiac Disease* was published in 1951. His research and recommendations were largely forgotten, until a parent, Elaine Gottschall, desperate to help her daughter, cured her daughter's illness using Dr. Haas's recommendations, and began helping thousands of others suffering from chronic gut issues as well as children with serious behavioral disorders.[10]

11. Vitamin and hormone deficiencies

Pyroluria is a severe deficiency in zinc, manganese, vitamin B6, and Omega 6 oils common in about 20 percent of autistic children.

Dr. David Brownstein reported resolving ADHD symptoms by treating iodine deficient hypothyroidism with a natural thyroid hormone replacement. He recommends checking basal body temperature before a child gets up in the morning, as a low temp signals a low functioning thyroid. Thyroid imbalance is more likely to occur during a large growth spurt, at menopause, during pregnancy, and at puberty. Dr. Brownstein also recommends sublingual Vitamin B12.

---

8   Dr. Natasha Campbell-McBride. *GAPS Gut and Psychology Syndrome.* 2012, pp. 314-315.
9   Association of family history of autoimmune diseases and autism spectrum disorders. *Pediatrics.* 2009 Aug;124(2):687-94.
10   Dr. Natasha Campbell-McBride. *GAPS Gut and Psychology Syndrome.* 2012, pp. 118-119.

12. Electromagnetic radiation

A study in the August, 2007 journal, *Australasian College of Nutritional & Environmental Medicine*, proposed that the electro-magnetic radiation (EMR) from wi-fi devices such as cell phones and routers interfere with the body's ability to clear toxins from the body – particularly heavy metals. Cells begin protecting themselves from the radiation, and a by-product is the retention of metals that should be excreted. When the vulnerable body of a child is then presented with heavy metals such as mercury in vaccinations or in some foods, then the inability to detoxify the cells causes a buildup of these heavy metals and interferes with normal brain processing resulting in the symptoms of autistic behavior.

13. GI Upset/Colic[11]

Children with autism are six to eight times more likely to suffer GI upset than children who are developing normally. Food allergies, leaky gut, type A blood, and lack of glutathione are predisposing factors. *Bacteroides fragilis* was recommended to treat leaky gut. Avoid gluten, dairy and soy.

14. Toxic load from endocrine disruptors

The body is exposed to toxins from cosmetics, toiletries, perfumes, and personal care products. The personal care product industry is not regulated, and many toxic substances are better absorbed through the skin than through the digestive system. One example is breast cancer. Cancerous breast cells are in many cases full of aluminum, which is the main ingredient of anti-perspirant deodorants. A pregnant woman passes toxins to the developing baby. Here are some of the most common toxins: talcum powder, sodium laurel sulfate (found in toothpaste), phthalates, chlorine, fluoride, titanium dioxide, DDT, saccharin, formaldehyde, propylene glycol, lead, aluminum and other toxic metals. Avoid BPA's in food cans and water bottles, fire retardants, and sulfates and xenoestrogens in personal care products.

15. Allergies and Asthma[12]

Researchers found that expectant mothers with asthma diagnosed in the second trimester were twice as likely to have a child that developed autism. The researchers found no risk among women found to have asthma during the third trimester.

The risk was smaller for women with allergies. The only significant effect was for women diagnosed with allergies in the second trimester. These women were 2.5 times as likely to have a child that developed autism.

16. Contraceptives and other drugs

Contraceptives have a devastating effect on the gut flora. Because a baby's gut is sterile when he is born, his mother passes on the abnormal gut to the child, predisposing the child to eczema, asthma, and other allergies, or more severe conditions. Other drugs also cause damage to the gut flora, including pain killers, steroids, sleeping pills, antacids, neuroleptics, and cholinolytic drugs. Drug-induced dysbiosis is the most severe, and most difficult to treat.

A 2012 study published in the journal *Pediatrics* warned that children's Tylenol may be associated with the increase in asthma. Acetaminophen reduces the body's supply of glutathione which is associated with oxidant damage in the lungs. Asthma has more than doubled since the 1970's

---

11 Gastrointestinal Problems in Children with Autism, Developmental Delays or Typical Development. *Journal of Autism and Developmental Disorders*, 6 November, 2013.

12 Allergies, Asthma May Play Role in Autism. Archives of *Pediatrics and Adolescent Medicine,* Feb. 2005.

when aspirin was replaced by Tylenol as the most common over the counter pain reliever for children. Very large studies have confirmed the association of Tylenol and asthma. In August 2010, the New York Times reported on data based on 322,000 children ages 13 and 14. Those who used acetaminophen once a month developed asthma symptoms twice as often as those who never take it. Between 1991 and 1993, the Boston University Fever Study gave 84,000 children low doses of acetaminophen or ibuprofen. For asthmatic children, the need for doctor's care was 2.3 times higher with Tylenol treatment than those treated with ibuprofen.

In February, 2014, the journal *JAMA Pediatrics* reported on a study of 64,000 children and mothers who took part in the Danish National Birth Cohort. The use of acetaminophen during pregnancy was associated with an increased risk of ADHD at age 7. The risk increased if Tylenol was taken in more than one trimester during pregnancy, and also increased the risk of cryptorchidism (undescended testis) in boys due to endocrine disruption. The study states, "Maternal hormones, such as sex hormones and thyroid hormones, play critical roles in regulating fetal brain development, and it is possible that acetaminophen may interrupt brain development by interfering with maternal hormones or via neurotoxicity."

17. Other linked conditions

Researchers from the University of Chicago published a study in March, 2014 linking male genital malformation with an increased incidence of autism. **Every 1% increase in malformations was linked to a 283% increase in autism.** A family history of early heart attacks is found in about 1/3 of families with an autistic child. Autistic children tend to have larger brains than other kids.

This chapter is meant to give you hope and resolve that you can optimize your children's health. You must act now to give your children all they need for the health and long life God intends for them to have. Slothful shopping for prepared junk foods, following a one-size-fits-all vaccine protocol, and ignoring toxins in our environment will have real life-long consequences for our children. Here is an action list you can implement today.

1. Commit your entire family to learning how to be fit for service in God's kingdom. You have learned how to eat clean and restore your health. Give your children the same gift. No excuses. No genetically modified food. We made this change with a resistant teenager. She came around. Eliminate wheat and dairy for 30 days, and see what it does for your family's health.

2. Take care of your largest detoxing organ, your skin. Do not put any chemicals on your skin that will increase toxins in your body. This includes mineral oil, propylene glycol, phthalates, sulfates, and dyes.

3. Use natural cleaning supplies, and avoid chemical pesticides. If your child has allergy symptoms, research further ways to make her room hypoallergenic.

4. You know your child best. Never vaccinate a sick child, even if the illness is mild. Give single vaccines only. Consider risk factors in making the vaccine decision that is right for you and your child. Exemption is your right to decide as a parent.

Measurements

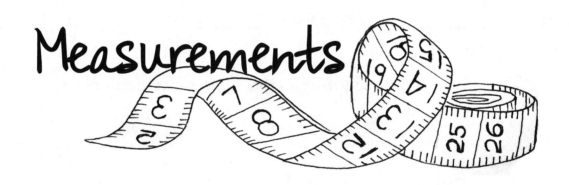

Day 11

Weight _____

Waist _____

2" Below _____

Hips _____

Thigh _____

Upper Arm _____

Day 18

Weight _____

Waist _____

2" Below _____

Hips _____

Thigh _____

Upper Arm _____

Day 25

Weight _____

Waist _____

2" Below _____

Hips _____

Thigh _____

Upper Arm _____

Be sure to measure in the same place each time.

Day 32

Weight _____

Waist _____

2" Below _____

Hips _____

Thigh _____

Upper Arm _____

Day 39

Weight _____

Waist _____

2" Below _____

Hips _____

Thigh _____

Upper Arm _____

Recipes

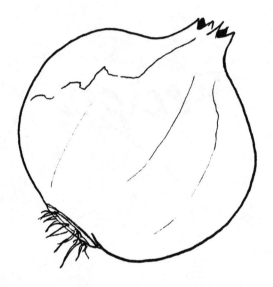

Salad Dressings

RECIPE	INGREDIENTS	DIRECTIONS
Avocado Mint Dressing	- 1 avocado - A few fresh mint leaves - 1 Tbsp balsamic vinaigrette - 1/2 cup roasted red peppers - water	Mix together all ingredients in a food processor except water. Slowly add water until creamy texture. Refrigerate.
Avocado Cilantro Dressing	- 1 avocado - 2 Tbsp cilantro - 1 tsp lemon juice - 1/2 tsp coriander - 1/2 tsp garlic - 1/2 tsp cumin - water	Mix together in a food processor. Pour water slowly until desired thickness.
Zesty French Dressing	- 1 small onion, chopped - 1/3 cup coconut milk - 1/3 cup balsamic vinegar - 4 grape tomatoes - 1 1/2 tsp soy sauce - 1 tsp salt - 1 tsp Dijon mustard - 1 Tbsp paprika - 1/2 tsp garlic powder - 1/2 tsp celery seed	Blend together all ingredients in a food processor. Blend until smooth and thickened. Refrigerate. Enjoy.
Toasted Almond Ginger Dressing	- 1/2 cup raw almonds - 1/2 cup unsweetened almond milk - 1 cup water - 6 pitted dates - 1 tsp garlic owder - 1 tsp. ginger - 1/2 yellow pepper	Blend well in a food processor and chill before serving.
Orange Honey Mustard Dressing	- 1/2 cup orange juice - 3 Tbsp honey - 2 Tbsp Dijon mustard - 1 1/2 cup water - 1 Tbsp non-GM cornstarch	In a small saucepan, mix all ingredients while cool. Heat on low until mixture thickens to a dressing consistency. Do not bring to a full boil.

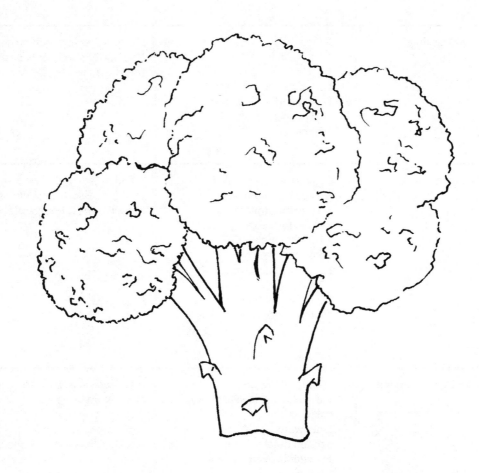

Salads and Soups

RECIPE	INGREDIENTS	DIRECTIONS
Edamame Salad	- 1 12 oz. pkg frozen shelled edamames - 1 cup frozen organic white corn - ¼ cup finely diced red onion - ½ red bell pepper - 2 Tbsp chopped cilantro - 1 Tbsp lemon juice - 1 tsp ginger - 2 Tbsp walnut oil - ¼ tsp fresh ground pepper	Mix all ingredients and refrigerate for a few hours before serving to let flavors blend.
Kale Salad	- ½ bunch of kale, chopped in a large food processor until fine - Add 2 each of celery, green onion and carrots, also chopped in the food processor - 1 avocado chopped by hand - 1 large tomato chopped by hand - 1 cup pine nuts or walnuts - 2 Tbsp lemon juice - 2 Tbsp walnut oil - 1 Tbsp Dijon mustard - Add stevia if you like a sweet cole slaw	
Spinach Salad	- ½ pound organic fresh spinach - 3 slices nitrate free bacon cooked crisp - 2 Tbsp coconut oil - ¼ cup balsamic vinegar - 2 Tbsp Dijon mustard - A few drops liquid stevia - Salt and pepper to taste	Cook over low heat until warm. Pour over spinach and sprinkle with bacon crumbs.
Quinoa Salad	- 2 cup quinoa, uncooked - 1/2 cup mushrooms - 1/2 cup fresh green beans - 1/2 cups carrots - 1/2 cup broccoli	Make quinoa according to package. Use half chicken stock and half water for more flavor. Steam vegetables until soft. Combine and toss together vegetables and quinoa. Serve warm.

Taco Salad	- 1 ½ pounds ground bison, organic beef or turkey - 1 Tbsp chili powder - ½ tsp garlic powder - ½ tsp cayenne pepper - ½ tsp oregano - 1½ tsp cumin - ½ tsp coriander	Simmer meat on low while chopping fresh ingredients for toppings: - Tomatoes - Green onions - Avocado - Refried or black beans - Red and yellow peppers - Sugar free salsa or pico de gallo Serve meat and toppings on a bed of romaine lettuce.
Chickpea Soup	- 1 15 oz can chickpeas, rinsed - 1 can coconut milk* - 1 cup chopped tomatoes - 1 chopped onion - 1 red pepper chopped - 1 small can green chilis - 1 tsp garlic powder - 1 qt. vegetable broth or chicken broth - 2 tsp curry powder	Bring to a boil and simmer until flavors are blended. *I recommend the Thai Kitchen brand.
Chickpea Soup 2	- 2 16 oz. cans garbanzo beans, rinsed and drained (read the label—no additives!) - 1 16 oz. can organic diced tomatoes - 1 diced red pepper - 1 medium onion chopped - 2 tsp cumin - ½ tsp cayenne pepper - ½ cup currants - 2 Tbsp almond butter	Simmer until flavors are blended together. Serve with 4 oz. organic meat and a mixed green salad.
Mexican Chicken Chowder	- ½ lb. boneless chicken breast - ½ cup chopped onions - 1 cup chicken or vegetable broth - 1 can coconut milk - 1 tsp garlic powder - 2 oz. green chilis - 5 fresh tomatoes - 1 can garbanzo beans - 1 tsp coriander - 1 tsp cumin - ¼ tsp baking soda - Optional: Salt and pepper to taste	Grill chicken and slice in ½ in. cubes. Use food processor to dice tomatoes. Combine all ingredients in a large pot. Simmer 15 minutes and enjoy!

Moroccan Chicken Soup	- 2 lbs boneless Chicken, cubed - 16 oz. jar sugar-free Salsa - 1 cup crushed pineapple, unsweetened - 1 diced orange - 1 cup water - 2 Tbsp honey - 2 tsp cumin - 1 tsp cinnamon	Combine all ingredients in a crock pot. Cook on high heat for four to six hours. After cooked, take a fork and shred chicken. Serve in a bowl on a bed of quinoa and cilantro. Enjoy!!
Orange Black Bean with Cumin Soup	- 2 (15-ounce) cans black beans, rinsed and drained - 1 green onion, minced - 1 rib celery, minced - 1/2 cup orange juice - 1/2 cup chicken broth - 1/2 tsp cumin - 1 dash cinnamon - Salt and Pepper to taste	Combine beans, shallot, celery, orange juice, broth, cumin, and cinnamon in a slow cooker. Cover and cook on high for about 1 1/2 hours. (Or on low for four to six hours). You can eat the soup on a bed of 1/2 cup Quinoa or brown rice, garnished with cilantro and fresh tomatoes.
Pumpkin Soup	- ½ chopped red pepper - ½ chopped large onion - 1 tsp dried parsley - ¼ tsp thyme - 1 bay leaf - 1 cup diced tomatoes - 1 lb. can pumpkin - 2 cups chicken stock - 1 cup coconut milk - 1 Tbsp non-GMO corn starch - 1 tsp sea salt - Fresh ground black pepper	Saute pepper, onion, and spices in 2 tsp. coconut oil until soft. Add remainder of ingredients except coconut milk and corn starch and stir well. Simmer 30 minutes. If you want smooth restaurant style soup, let cool and run through a food processor or blender. Return to pan and add coconut milk and corn starch. Bring to a careful boil, stirring frequently. Serve immediately.
Seafood Soup	- 46 oz. organic chicken broth - 6 oz. organic carrots finely chopped - ¼ head cabbage - 1 large onion - 4 stalks celery - 2 turnips - 4 oz. fresh mushrooms - 1 pound cooked shrimp chopped - 6 oz. crab meat - 2 Tbsp Old Bay Seasoning - ½ tsp black pepper - 1 can coconut milk	Combine all ingredients and simmer until carrots are tender, about ½ hour.

Fresh Tomato Soup	- ¼ cup cold pressed organic coconut oil - 1 medium chopped onion - ¼ cup non GMO corn starch - 4 large fresh tomatoes, pureed in food processer - 4 cups coconut milk (from the half gallon carton in refrigerator section) - 1 15 oz can organic tomato sauce - 1 tsp Italian seasoning - ½ tsp black pepper - ½ tsp baking soda	Saute chopped onion in coconut oil until soft. Add the rest of the ingredients and simmer 10 minutes. Serve with a salad that contains protein—sliced eggs, black beans, almonds; or a quinoa salad.
Basic Vegetable Soup	- 1 cup diced carrots - 1 large onion - 2 stalks celery - ¼ head cabbage - 1 cup green beans - 1 chopped yellow squash - 1 28 oz. can diced tomatoes - 48 oz. vegetable broth - 1 tsp cumin - 2 cups water - 1 can kidney or pinto beans rinsed (organic, or check to make sure they are sugar free and in a BPA free can) - Salt and pepper.	Simmer about 20 minutes and serve.

Snacks and Sides

RECIPE	INGREDIENTS	DIRECTIONS
Deviled Eggs	- 6 eggs - 3 cups water - Pinch of salt - 1 medium avocado - 3 Tbsp Dijon mustard - Paprika to sprinkle	Place eggs, water and salt into medium saucepan. Water should just cover your eggs. Bring to a boil. Boil for 10 minutes, remove from heat. Drain, and refill with cool water. Allow eggs to cool. Peel and half eggs. Remove egg yolks from egg white. Place all yokes into a medium sized bowl. Beat together egg yolk, avocado, and mustard until smooth. Divide yolk mixture evenly among egg halves and sprinkle with paprika.
Protein Bars	- 4 cups vanilla protein powder - ¼ cup almond butter - 15 oz. coconut milk - 1 tsp almond extract	Mix by hand or in a large food processor. Press into a 9 x 13 pan and refrigerate at least 1 hour. Cut into 20 bars, 75 calories each. These can be wrapped individually and frozen so you can grab and go. Enjoy with a large Granny Smith apple, sliced into 16 pieces and sprinkled with stevia and cinnamon.
Sweet Potato Fries	- 1-2 sweet potatoes - Coconut oil - Stevia - Cinnamon	Cover a cookie sheet with aluminum foil and rub with coconut oil. Slice sweet potatoes into fries and spread one layer deep until cookie sheet is covered. Sprinkle with stevia and cinnamon. Place in 425 degree oven until fries are soft, about 20 minutes depending on thickness.

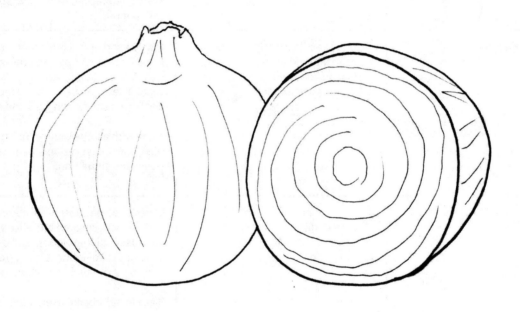

Main Dish

RECIPE	INGREDIENTS	DIRECTIONS
Burgers on the Grill	- 1 lb. organic lean ground beef or turkey - ½ cup almond meal - 1/3 cup tomato sauce - 1 medium onion - ½ tsp.garlic powder - 1 egg - Salt and pepper to taste	Mix thoroughly and form patties to cook on the grill. The Against All Grains website has a recipe for hamburger buns that are grain free! But, if you are counting calories, eat it with a lettuce wrap topped with sugar free salsa, Dijon mustard, or a fresh tomato slice, and serve with lots of green vegetables.
Coconut Curry	- 1 serving - 4 oz boneless organic chicken - 1/2 cup almond milk - 1 tsp curry powder - 1/2 cup coconut milk - 1 Tbsp rice flour - 1 small diced onion - 2 Tbsp unsweetened coconut - 1/4 green apple, cubed - 1/2 cup brown rice	Cook brown rice according to bag. Place chicken and diced onion in a small pan. Cover and let simmer until chicken is cooked through. Add almond milk, coconut milk, rice flour (for thickening), and curry powder on medium heat. Cook until sauce is thickened. Pour into a bowl over brown rice. Sprinkle with unsweetened coconut and green apple. Serve with a large salad.
Chicken and No Dumplings	- 2-3 lb. boneless skinless Chicken breasts - 1 large onion - 4-5 stalks celery - 1 lb mini carrots - 1 large red pepper - 1 large yellow pepper - 1 cup coconut milk - 1 cup almond milk - 3 Tbsp organic corn starch	Grill chicken for five minutes on each side to add flavor and cook out fat. Cut into 2 inch pieces and place in large crock pot. Add chopped onion, chopped celery, and halved mini-carrots. Add 2 cups water, salt to taste and allow cooking until carrots are tender and chicken is done. Remove meat and vegetables and pour juice into 2 quart sauce pan. Add 1 cup coconut milk, 1 cup almond milk with 3 Tbsp organic cornstarch stirred in before adding to juice. Let simmer until thickened. Serve half as gravy, and pour other half over vegetables and meat. Can be served over brown rice or quinoa.

Chicken Stir Fry	**Marinade:** - 2 Tbsp Braggs Aminos - ½ tsp ginger - Dash of garlic - 1 packet stevia **Vegetables:** - 1 medium onion sliced - 2 stalks celery sliced - 1 red or yellow bell pepper sliced - 1 large tomato cut in wedges **Sauce:** - 2 Tbsp walnut oil - 1 packet stevia - 2 Tbsp Braggs Aminos - 2 Tbsp non GMO corn starch - 1 cup water	Cut up two pounds organic boneless chicken breasts into 1 inch cubes and marinate for 30 min and up to overnight. Brown meat in 2 Tbsp walnut oil and set aside Cook the vegetables for two to three minutes. Add chicken. Mix sauce and boil one minute. Pour over meat and vegetables and serve with quinoa, if desired.
Hawaiian Chicken	- 2 lbs boneless chicken breasts - 1 cup orange juice - ¼ cup soy sauce - 1 tsp ginger - ¼ tsp pepper - 1 medium onion - 1 can pineapple chunks, in unsweetened juice	Combine all ingredients in a crock pot on high heat for three hours. Serve with ½ cup quinoa or rice, cooked according to package.
Lemon Ginger Chicken	- 6 boneless skinless chicken breasts - 1/2 cup almond flour - 1/4 cup egg white - Powdered organic ginger - Lemon pepper - Garlic	Preheat oven to 400 degrees. In one bowl pour egg white. In another bowl mix almond flour, and a dash of ginger, lemon pepper, and garlic. Take each piece of chicken and dip in egg white, and then into almond flour mixture. Place chicken in a 9x13 in pan. Repeat with each chicken breast. Bake in oven for 50 minutes or until tender when cut. Enjoy with a large portion of steamed vegetables.
Thai Chicken	- 4 boneless chicken breasts - 3 Tbsp walnut oil **Seasoning:** - 1 tsp. garlic powder - ½ tsp. ginger **Sauce:** - ¼ cup Braggs Aminos (soy sauce alternative) - 3 Tbsp almond butter - 1 Tbsp apple cider vinegar - ¼ cup water	Saute chicken until cooked through. Chop into 1 inch cubes. Add seasoning and toss. Mix sauce and pour over chicken. Let simmer for a few minutes. You can add fresh vegetables such as broccoli, sugar snap peas, onions, and cauliflower the last five minutes.

Homemade Chili	- 1 lb. organic ground beef or bison - ½ cup onion, diced - 1 can diced tomatoes - 1 can tomato paste - 1 cup water - 1½ can of tomato sauce - 2 cans dark red kidney beans - 2 tsp chili powder - 1 tsp cayenne pepper - 1 tsp basil - 1 tsp Italian seasoning	Buy organic grass fed beef. Brown ground beef in a skillet with onions. Pat with paper towel after cooking to remove excess oil. Combine all ingredients in a large frying pan. Bring to a boil, reduce heat to low and cover. Let simmer. Check tomato products and beans—no sugar, no MSG! It's amazing what they add sugar to. Read every label. Costco sells organic tomatoes, sauce, and paste for less than non-organics at the grocery. Organic is always the right choice!
White Chili	- 1 lb. white northern beans, soaked overnight in cold water and drained - 6 cups chicken broth - 2 cups coconut milk - 2 tsp garlic powder - 1 large onion chopped - 1 lb. boneless skinless chicken - 8 oz. green chiles - 1 chopped jalapeno pepper without seeds - 2 tsp Italian seasoning - 2 tsp ground cumin - ½ tsp allspice - ½ tsp cayenne pepper - 1 tsp chili pepper - 4 Tbsp chopped fresh cilantro - 1 tsp sea salt	Brown the chicken over medium heat and cut into small cubes. Add all ingredients to a 2 gallon soup pot and simmer over low heat around 6 hours.
Pot Roast	- Choose a brisket or lean cut of organic beef. - 1 cup beef broth - 2 Tbsp coconut oil - Carrots, chopped - Turnips - Cabbage - Salt & pepper to taste	Sprinkle with salt and pepper. Brown on all sides in a frying pan in 2 Tbsp coconut oil. Place in a crock pot and add carrots, turnips, cabbage, and 1 cup beef broth. Cook for 6-8 hours or until tender. Remember 4 oz. of lean meat is a good serving of protein. We have changed our understanding of portions. Fill your plate with salad and fresh green vegetables.
Grilled Salmon	- Wild caught salmon fillet - 3 Tbsp soy sauce - 3 Tbsp lemon juice - 3 packets stevia natural sweetener - 1 tsp Coconut Oil - Aluminum Foil	Marinate salmon in a baking pan with soy sauce, lemon juice and stevia for 30 minutes. Put coconut oil on a sheet of aluminum foil and place on the heated grill. Cook salmon meat side down for five minutes, then flip to skin side down until done. Skin will stick to foil, and fish can be cut in servings and picked up with a spatula.

| Veggie Burgers | - 1 lb organic baby carrots
- 4 stalks celery
- 1/2 head of cauliflower
- 1/2 cup sesame seeds
- 1 lg onion
- 1/2 red bell pepper
- 1 tsp basil
- 1 tsp oregano
- 1 tsp parsley
- 1/2 cup flax seed meal
- 1 tsp salt
- 1 tsp garlic powder
- 1/3 cup almond meal
- 1 tsp black pepper
- 1 egg | In a large pot add 2 cups water and a vegetable steamer. Add carrots, cauliflower and celery. Steam until soft, about 15 minutes. Transfer half of mixture to a food processor and puree with the chopping blade. Repeat with second half. Add sesame seeds to processor and blend. Place pureed food in a large mixing bowl and set aside.
In a medium frying pan saute onions and pepper in 1 tsp coconut oil until soft. Add parsley, oregano and basil. Combine well and add to mixing bowl.

Add remaining ingredients and mix well. Cover baking sheet with aluminum foil and lightly spray with olive oil spray. Using a 1/4 cup measuring cup spoon mixture onto baking sheet and press patty until 3/4 in thick.

Bake at 375 ° for fifteen minutes on each side, or until golden brown. Enjoy!! |
| **White Fish with Quinoa Stuffing** | - 3-4 white fish filets
- 1 cup quinoa, rinsed
- 1 cup celery, diced
- 1 cup sweet onion, diced
- 1 cup chicken or vegetable broth
- 2 tsp poultry seasoning
- 2 eggs
- ½ cup almond milk | Slice each filet into two layers so it can be stuffed.

Cook 1 cup quinoa by boiling in 2 cups water, or 1 cup water, 1 cup chicken stock.

In a frying pan rubbed with coconut oil, add 1 cup chopped sweet onion, 1 cup celery. Cover with lid and let simmer 5 minutes until soft. Turn off the burner. Add poultry seasoning and cooked quinoa. Let cool slightly. Beat two eggs and almond milk with a fork and add to quinoa. Fill each fish with stuffing, and set the rest around the filets in a 9x13 pan.

Bake 20 minutes at 425 degrees or until fish is flaky and done. Fish may be sprinkled with paprika for a garnish. |

References

Paula Baillie-Hamilton, M.D. *Toxic Overload, A Doctor's Plan for Combating the Illnesses Caused by Chemicals in our Foods, our Homes, and our Medicine Cabinets.* New York: Avery Publishing, 2005.

Sharon Batt. *Patient No More: The Politics of Breast Cancer.* Prince Edward Island, Canada: Gynergy Books, 1994.

Kenneth Bock, M.D. and Cameron Stauth. *Healing the New Childhood Epidemics: Autism, ADHD, Asthma and Allergies.* New York: Balantine Books, 2008.

Lee Bueno-Aquer. *Fast Your Way to Health.* New Kensington, PA: Whitaker House, 1991.

Dr. Natasha Campbell-McBride. *Gut and Psychology Syndrome.* 2012, 7th ed.. ISBN 978-0954852023.

Brian Clement. *Living Foods for Optimal Health.* Roseville, CA: Prima Publishing, 1996.

Dr. Don Colbert. *Walking in Divine Health.* Lake Mary, FL: Siloam Press, 1998.

Dr. Don Colbert. *Toxic Relief, Restore Health and Energy through Fasting and Detoxification.* Lake Mary, FL: Siloam Press, 2001.

Loren Cordain, Ph.D. *The Dietary Cure for Acne.* Fort Collins: Paleo Diet Enterprises, 2006.

William Davis, M.D. *Wheat Belly.* New York: Rodale Books, 2011.

Michael R. Eades, M.D. and Mary Dan Eades, M.D. *Protein Power: The High-Protein/Low-Carbohydrate Way to Lose Weight, Feel Fit, and Boost Your Health – In Just Weeks!* New York: Bantam Books, 1999.

Joseph Glenmullen, M.D. *The Antidepressant Solution: A Step-by-Step Guide to Safely Overcoming Antidepressant Withdrawal, Dependence, and "Addiction."* New York: Simon and Schuster, 2005.

Dallas and Melissa Hartwig. *It Starts with Food.* Las Vegas: Victory Belt Publishing, 2012.

Richard Hobday. *The Healing Sun.* Scotland: Findhorn Press, 1999.

The Holy Bible, King James Version. Public Domain.

Mark Hyman, M.D. and Mark Liponis, M.D. *Ultra-Prevention: The Six Week Plan That Will Make You Healthier For Life.* New York: Simon and Schuster, 2003.

Mark Hyman, M.D. *The Ultra-Metabolism Cookbook.* New York: Scribner, 2007.

Linda Jeffrey. *Comfort and Joy: How to Receive Healing Beyond Grief and Loss.* Crestwood: First Principles Press, 2012.

Alejandro Junger, M.D. *Clean Gut.* New York: Harper Collins, 2013.

Chris Kahlenborn, M.D. *Breast Cancer, Its Link to Abortion and the Birth Control Pill.* Dayton, OH: One More Soul Publishing, 2000.

David Kessler, M.D. *The End of Overeating. Taking Control of the Insatiable American Appetite.* New York: Rodale Press, 2009.

John and Sheila Kippley. *The Art of Natural Family Planning.* Cincinnati: The Couple to Couple League International, 3rd ed., 1991.

Dr. John Lee and David Zava, Ph.D. *What Your Doctor May Not Tell You About Breast Cancer.* New York: Time Warner, 2002.

Dr. John Lee. *What Your Doctor May Not Tell You About Pre-menopause.* New York: Warner Books, 2004.

John R. Lee, M.D., *Hormone Balance for Men: What Your Doctor May Not Tell You About Prostate Health and Natural Hormone Supplementation.* Dr. Lee cites the work of Dr. Calavieri reported in 1998 by the National Cancer Institute and available as NCI Monograph #27 from Oxford University Press.

Dr. John Lee and Virginia Warner. *What Your Doctor May Not Tell You About Menopause.* New York: Warner Books, 2004.

Janet Maccaro, Ph.D. *90 Day Immune System Makeover.* Lake Mary, FL: Siloam Press, 2000.

Kathryn Marsden. *Good Gut Bugs, How the healing power of probiotics can transform your health.* London: Piatkus Publishing, 2010.

S. I. McMillen, M.D. *None of These Diseases.* Zenda, WI: Pyramid Publishing, 1963.

Christiane Northrup, M.D. *The Wisdom of Menopause.* New York: Bantam Books, 2001.

Deanna Osborn and Linda Jeffrey. *Dr. Deanna's Healing Handbook.* Crestwood: First Principles Press, 2014.

Christian Overman. *Assumptions that Affect Our Lives.* Simi Valley: Micah 6:8 Publishing, 1996.

Lester Packer, Ph. D. *The Antioxidant Miracle.* New York: John Wiley & Sons, 1999.

Leanne Payne. *The Broken Image, Restoring Personal Wholeness through Healing Prayer.* Wheaton, IL: Crossway Books, 1981.

Nicholas Perricone, M.D. *The Wrinkle Cure.* New York: Warner Books, 2001.

Nicholas Perricone, M.D. *The Perricone Prescription and Personal Journal.* New York: Warner Books, 2002.

Nicholas Perricone, M.D. *The Perricone Promise.* New York: Warner Books, 2004.

David Perlmutter, M.D. and Carol Colman. *The Better Brain Book.* New York: Riverhead Books, 2004.

David Perlmutter, M.D. and Kristin Loberg. *Grain Brain: The Surprising Truth about Wheat, Carbs, and Sugar—Your Brain's Silent Killers.* New York: Little, Brown and Co., 2013.

Michael Pollan. *Cooked, A Natural History of Transformation.* New York: Penguin Press, 2013.

Charles D. Provan. *The Bible and Birth Control.* Monongahela, PA: Zimmer Printing, 1989.

Sherry A. Rogers, M.D. *Detoxify or Die.* Sarasota, FL: Sand Key Company, 2002.

Ron Rosedale, M.D. with Carol Coleman. *The Rosedale Diet.* New York: Harper Collins, 2004.

Joel Salatin. *Folks, This Ain't Normal.* New York: Hachette Book Group, 2011.

Ted Schettler, M.D. *In Harms Way: Toxic Threats to Child Development.* Boston Physicians for Social Responsibility, 2000. <http://psr.lgc.org/ihwrept/ihwcomplete.pdf>

Barbara Seaman. *The Greatest Experiment Ever Performed on Women: Exploding the Estrogen Myth.* New York: Hyperion Books, 2003.

Suzanne Somers. *Breakthrough, Eight Steps to Wellness.* New York: Crown Publishers, 2008.

Toni Weschler. *Taking Charge of Your Fertility: The Definitive Guide to Natural Birth Control, Pregnancy Achievement, and Reproductive Health.* New York: Harper Collins, 2002

James Wilson. *Adrenal Fatigue – The 21st Century Stress Syndrome.* Petaluma, CA: Smart Publications, 2001.

www.AppetiteforGod.com